A WORLD BANK COUNTRY STUDY

West Bank and Gaza

*Medium-Term Development Strategy
for the Health Sector*

The World Bank
Washington, D.C.

World Bank Country Studies are among the many reports originally prepared for internal use as part of the continuing analysis by the Bank of the economic and related conditions of its developing member countries and of its dialogues with the governments. Some of the reports are published in this series with the least possible delay for the use of governments and the academic, business and financial, and development communities. The typescript of this paper therefore has not been prepared in accordance with the procedures appropriate to formal printed texts, and the World Bank accepts no responsibility for errors. Some sources cited in this paper may be informal documents that are not readily available.

ISSN: 0253-2123

Library of Congress Cataloging-in-Publication Data

West Bank and Gaza : medium-term development strategy for the health
    sector.
        p.   cm. — (A World Bank country study)
    Includes bibliographical references (p.).
    ISBN 0-8213-4230-4
    1. Medical policy—West Bank.   2. Medical policy—Gaza Strip.
   3. Medical care—West Bank.   4. Medical care—Gaza Strip.
   5. Medical economics—West Bank.   6. Medical economics—Gaza Strip.
   I. World Bank.   II. Series.
   RA395.W47W47   1998
   362.1'095695'3—dc21
                                    98-12237
                                    CIP

CONTENTS

APPENDICES

This report is based on the findings of a mission which visited West Bank and Gaza in May 1997. This report is the work of the MOH, World Bank and WHO. The MOH team was led by H.E. Dr. Riyad Zanoun (Minister of Health and Head of the Policy Planning Committee) and Dr. Munzer Sharif (Deputy Minister). The World Bank team included: Egbe Osifo (Task Manager), Atsuko Aoyama (Health Specialist), Jan Bultman (Health Insurance Specialist), Ernst Lauridsen (Pharmaceutical Specialist), Akiko Maeda (Health Financing Specialist), Isabelle Schnadig (Economist), Philippe Schpereel (Hospital Management Specialist) and Shehla Zaidi (Health Specialist). Ali Khadr (Deputy Resident Representative) provided macroeconomic advice. Nigel Roberts (HQ Manager) provided NGO advice. The WHO team consisted of Dr. Paolo Piva (Resident Coordinator), Mr. Joseph Hazbun (Senior Adviser, Emergency Humanitarian Assistance Division) and Dr. Othman Karameh (Medical Officer). The study team would like to acknowledge UNRWA, Palestinian Bureau of Statistics and other agencies and individuals for the information and insight they provided during the preparation of this report. The peer reviewers were Messrs. Willy De Geydnt and Jack Langenbunner. The report was formatted by Vivian Nwachukwu and Karine Pezzani, MNSHD. The Sector Director is Mr. Jacques Baudouy and the Country Director is Mr. Joseph Saba.

Foreword

When I had a heart attack while reading the concluding remarks for this study, I thought it had just been the excitement mixed with the satisfaction brought about by the hard work of all parties and the outcome of this very important event.

Now, after my recovery and coming back to continue our health developmental march, the first thing I thought to do was write this foreword to highlight the unique situation of this work which presents a model of how the West Bank and Gaza, represented by the Ministry of Health, is working hand in hand with World Health Organization and the World Bank. I feel so proud of all that has been done by the International and Local experts who met together to exchange ideas and choose the best available alternative to achieve health for people.

Before the final version was completed, this report had been tackled with great concern by the Ministry of Health, to the extent that immediate steps for health reform were put into action. The Ministry of Health is following the report's advice regarding maximizing utilization of the available beds in government hospitals and sub-contracting with non governmental organizations and private health facilities. The large figure of expenditures for overseas referrals had been reduced by 35% during 1997.

The situation in Palestine is dynamic with continuous changes that are difficult to predict. The last Palestinian population census showed that we have to make planning a continuous dynamic process. The total population exceeds our previous expectations and is now 3.1 million inhabitants. A second example of the frequent changes is the difference between our expectations of US$27 million in health insurance premiums and the US$50 million achieved in extremely difficult circumstances. The percentage of Insured Families reached 48%.

These dynamic changes have necessitated the attachment of relevant updated data.

Finally, we have to extend our deep thanks to the great determination, commitment and dedication showed by each and every participant in this serious but realistic and well coordinated effort.

Riyad Zanoun
Minister of Health

ABSTRACT

West Bank and Gaza's health system is at an evolutionary crossroads. Its improvement will depend largely on the Ministry of Health's ability to mobilize political support among various stakeholders, including policymakers, consumers, care providers, the legislative council and donors. The Ministry also faces the challenge of developing a coherent health strategy to cover a divided geographical area in a complex political and economic situation. The issues this challenge presents are unique and difficult.

This report – a joint product of the Palestinian Authority, the World Bank and the World Health Organization – assesses the performance and prospects of the health sector in West Bank–Gaza, providing a focal point for an ongoing development dialogue. Its analysis of sector delivery, financing and governance suggests the following short and medium term actions: (a) ensure financial sustainability by reevaluating the public investment plan in light of revised macroeconomic projections; (b) improve efficiency through sector wide initiatives; (c) improve the quality of services provided by improving delivery processes; and (d) clarify the roles and responsibilities of various sector agencies, with a focus on strengthening the Ministry's role in regulatory and policy functions and improving its insurance operations, as well as those at the Government Health Insurance organization.

CURRENCY EQUIVALENTS
Currency Unit = New Israeli Shekel (NIS)
Currency Unit = Jordanian Dinar (JD)

EXCHANGE RATE AS OF JUNE 1997
NIS 1.00 = US$0.29
US$1.00 = NIS 3.52
JD 1.00 = US$1.49
US$1.00 = JD 0.71

WEST BANK AND GAZA FISCAL YEAR
January 1 - December 31

LIST OF ACRONYMS

BSN	Baccalaureate Degree of Nursing
GHI	Government Health Insurance
GMP	Good Manufacturing Practices
GNP	Gross National Product
GDP	Gross Domestic Product
IEC	Information, Education and Communication
IMR	Infant Mortality Rate
JMA	Jordanian Medical Association
MENA	Middle East and North Africa
MOH	Ministry of Health
MRIs	Magnetic Resonance Imagers
NGOs	Nongovernmental Organizations
NIS	New Israeli Shekel
PA	Palestinian Authority
PHC	Primary Health Care
PRCS	Palestine Red Crescent Society
QIP	Quality Improvement Program
TBA	Traditional Birth Attendant
UNRWA	United Nations Relief and Work Agency for Palestine Refugees in the Near East
WBG	West Bank and Gaza
WHO	World Health Organization

EXECUTIVE SUMMARY

INTRODUCTION

This report, a joint effort of the Ministry of Health (MOH), World Bank and WHO, provides the MOH with short to medium term policy recommendations designed to ensure the financial sustainability of the health sector while improving access to health care as well as its efficiency and quality.

The West Bank and Gaza (WBG) is comprised of two geographically separated areas with a combined population currently at 2.3 million and growing at 3.7 percent per annum. The WBG, a lower middle income economy, has a GNP per capita of US$1,710.[1] Compared to other lower middle income countries, the Palestinian population is well educated (84 percent literacy) and their overall health status is relatively good (*e.g.,* IMR is 28 per 1,000 live births).

PROBLEMS

The impressive health and education status now enjoyed in WBG may not be sustainable. Severe economic disruptions related to the extremely complex political situation have caused the macroeconomic environment to deteriorate: per capita incomes fell by 7 percent in 1996 alone, unemployment is estimated at least at 30 percent and about one fifth of the population is estimated to live in poverty. The deteriorating economic environment can influence health status through rising poverty (the poor are less healthy) and by constraining expenditures on health and education.

The financial sustainability of currently planned investments provides a good illustration of this latter problem. In 1994,

---

[1] World Bank estimates, using the Atlas methodology. However, the purchasing power of one dollar within the WBG is likely to be influenced by its close links to the much richer Israeli economy and rising inflation (8 percent in 1996).

the National Health Plan was prepared with an assumption that economic growth would be relatively stable and with a goal of rapid health system expansion. In 1997, when many of the planned investments are about to become operational, resources available to operate them are declining. By 2002, estimates place the annual cost associated with operating all planned new facilities at over 25 percent of the total MOH budget. Financial sustainability of all sector activities – not just of investments – is further threatened by rising drug expenditure. Pharmaceuticals are the fastest growing component of MOH's recurrent budget, increasing from 22 percent of total health expenditure in 1995 to a projected 32 percent of expenditure in 1997.

While investment planning assumptions affect the prospects for sustainability, the current organization of the system presents other problems. Overall sectoral efficiency could be improved, as shown in the varying utilization rates, with for instance 83 percent of capacity at use in MOH hospitals, compared to 64 percent in NGO hospitals. At the same time, the perception of both providers and patients is that the quality of health services could be enhanced. While most of the population has reasonable physical access to health facilities, effective financial access is constrained for the one half of all households which is not covered by the health insurance program - Government Health Insurance (GHI) -. These households must bear, in out of pocket payments at the time of illness, the full cost of health care. Many of these households may have chosen to opt out of the GHI. Anecdotal evidence however suggests that others such as the non-refugee poor have not done so voluntarily and yet face great financial difficulties in accessing health care. This raises concerns about the effectiveness of the government's social welfare program, which is supposed to fully cover the indigent population's GHI premiums. UNRWA, which is currently facing major financial problems, is responsible for the provision of basic care to registered refugees.

RECOMMENDATIONS

The challenges facing the MOH in its attempt to develop a coherent health strategy to cover a divided geographical area in a complex political situation are unique and difficult. The recent economic downturn exacerbates the difficulties. Inaction however will result only in further deterioration of the system and the health status of the population. This report offers a number of suggestions for short and medium term actions to improve the situation.

Ensure that the system is financially sustainable

Reevaluation of the affordability and sustainability of the public investment strategy is urgently needed. At the same time, immediate action is also needed to contain recurrent costs in critical areas including drug expenditure and overseas treatment. Pharmaceutical reforms could reduce drug expenditures by 30 to 40 percent of their present level.

Improve efficiency through sector wide initiatives

Employing strategies to increase the efficiency and effectiveness of resource use will require an improved understanding of financial flows, utilization patterns and demand for services in all sub-sectors. This information can be used to design measures under the following three broad strategies, each of which would result in significant efficiency gains.

- Improve the delivery system's technical efficiency by strengthening facility level management capacity.

- Strengthen the role of primary care givers and improve the referral system.

- Increase the complementarity of government, private and NGO services.

Measures designed to pursue these strategies will also require staged development of a provider payment system conducive to cost containment and the capacity to contract between MOH/GHI and various NGO/private providers and to monitor provider performance under these contracts. Improving sectoral management information systems will thus be crucial to efficiency improvement efforts.

The gains to be had from improving sector efficiency are large. If, for example, the average occupancy rate of the hospital beds reaches 80 percent, the cost of the proposed public investment plan could be reduced by at least US$63 million. This would in turn reduce the recurrent costs needed to operate the new facilities investments by about US$32 million each year.

Improve the quality of services provided

Improving the processes involved in delivery should be the first focus of quality improvement measures. Protocols and standards for medical procedures need to be established and integrated into various training programs. Similar protocols and standards should be gradually introduced in MOH and UNRWA facilities. Uniform licensing for all health professionals should be required and could be used to spur demand for continuing education among professionals. This would also contribute to harmonizing the level of professional competence of health care providers. A sustainable human resource strategy for the sector should be developed. Improved planning and training of the health work-force however will not by itself improve patient care; it must also be accompanied by work conditions (including salaries and non-financial remuneration) which motivate professionals in the sector to provide quality services.

The role and responsibilities of various agencies (including MOH) within the sector should be better defined, and should form part of a unified regulatory framework.

The MOH needs to strengthen its role in regulatory and policy functions, and to improve the insurance function of MOH/GHI. Immediate steps could be taken to strengthen MOH's revenue collection capacity. Mobilizing employers contribution through group contracts would be a reasonable first step in this regard.

In the longer term, the government needs to decide on its chosen option towards achieving universal financial access for health care.

CONCLUSION

WBG is at a crossroads in the evolution of its health system. The prospects for improving the health system depend largely on the ability of the MOH to mobilize sufficient political support among various stakeholders (including key policy-makers, consumers, providers, the legislative council and donor agencies) to implement the changes proposed in this report. The process of developing the new National Health Plan will provide an opportunity to foster a policy dialogue and to build consensus. This will help ensure that the necessary political support materializes. Donors can help in two main ways. They can support capacity building in management, policy formulation and service delivery that would result in the development of sustainable local institutions, and they can provide financial assistance to those investments which are financially sustainable within the limits of WBG resources in the medium to long term. Together, these measures will engender an effective and efficient health delivery system.

This report attempts to provide a focal point for ongoing dialogue in the sector. The World Bank and WHO stand ready to assist in facilitating a process of review and discussion by Palestinian constituencies and the donor community. It has to be recognized that the Palestinian health sector is not static, and the MOH has already started implementing several of the recommendations included in this report during the course of its preparation. Whatever answers are ultimately adopted by WBG authorities, the strategic issues identified in this report will have a significant impact on the Palestinian health system in the years to come.

1. BACKGROUND

INTRODUCTION

The Palestinian Authority (PA) is facing extremely difficult economic and political challenges as it tries to develop policies to lead the transformation of the Palestinian economy into a globally-oriented, market-based economy. Human capital development - which includes improving health status - is a key factor in ensuring sustainable economic development. The PA is taking steps to ensure that previous gains in health status are not compromised; and that the health sector develops the capacity to play an important role in developing the main Palestinian resource - its people.

Consequently, this joint effort by the MOH, the World Bank and WHO will assess the sector and suggest a medium term strategy that could help the PA achieve its objectives. It will assess the health sector in terms of: (a) efficiency and quality of services; (b) sustainability of present financial arrangements; and (c) equity and accessibility to services. It provides the MOH with policy recommendations to ensure financial sustainability while improving efficiency, quality and access to health care. The study concludes with suggested public financing priorities for the short to medium term and identifies possible areas in which the World Bank, WHO, and other interested donors might be able to assist the PA in the future. This report is complemented by technical background papers in health financing, reproductive health, pharmaceuticals and health insurance which are available in a separate volume.

The report complements recent World Bank economic and sector work, primarily the multisectoral economic report "The West Bank and Gaza: Economic Report" and the work financed under the health component of the Technical Assistance Trust Fund administered by the World Bank. It also complements on-going work on the five-year

health plan being developed by the PA. The study draws on data from available sources and reports from the MOH and other PA agencies including the Palestinian Central Bureau of Statistics, United Nations agencies, WHO, the World Bank and other relevant organizations. Other sources of information included direct interviews with local responsible personnel and clients and field visits.

ECONOMIC AND POLITICAL BACKGROUND

The West Bank and Gaza (WBG) comprises two geographically separated areas with a combined area of 6,000 square kilometers. The 1996 estimated population was about 2.3 million, of which about 65 percent reside in the West Bank. Registered refugees represent about a quarter of the West Bank population and two thirds of Gaza Strip population. The population is young (47 percent is under 15 years) and growing rapidly at 3.7 percent per year.

The West Bank and Gaza Strip differ in terms of natural landscape, population distribution and legal heritage. The West Bank population is dispersed among 422 towns, villages and camps at a population density of 267 persons per square kilometer compared with Gaza Strip where the population is concentrated into 16 towns, villages and camps with a population density of 2,596 persons per square kilometer. In Gaza Strip, about half of the refugee population lives in camps compared to about a quarter in the West Bank. Historically Gaza Strip was administered by Egypt while the West Bank was administered by Jordan, and this difference is still reflected in their respective legal regimes. The WBG had a GNP per capita of US$1,710 in 1996,[2] which categorizes it as a lower-middle

---

[2] World Bank estimates, using the Atlas methodology. However the purchasing power of one dollar within the WBG is likely to be influenced by its close links to the much richer Israeli economy and rising inflation (8 percent in 1996).

income economy. GNP per capita in Gaza Strip is half of that of the West Bank. Between 1993 and 1996, there has been a deterioration in economic conditions. These may be explained, to a large extent, by the tumultuous socio-political and economic environment which has proved to be far less positive and less predictable than initially anticipated. For example:

Although recent data on output and incomes in the WBG remain sparse and incomplete, tentative estimates suggested that real GNP per capita (which, in addition to domestic output takes account of income earned abroad) fell sharply in the WBG by about 7 percent in 1996 alone. The unemployment rate[4] was estimated to be about 28 percent in 1996[5] compared to 11 percent in 1993. The dire macroeconomic situation is

Figure 1: Impact of the Closures on Monthly Health Insurance Premium Revenues

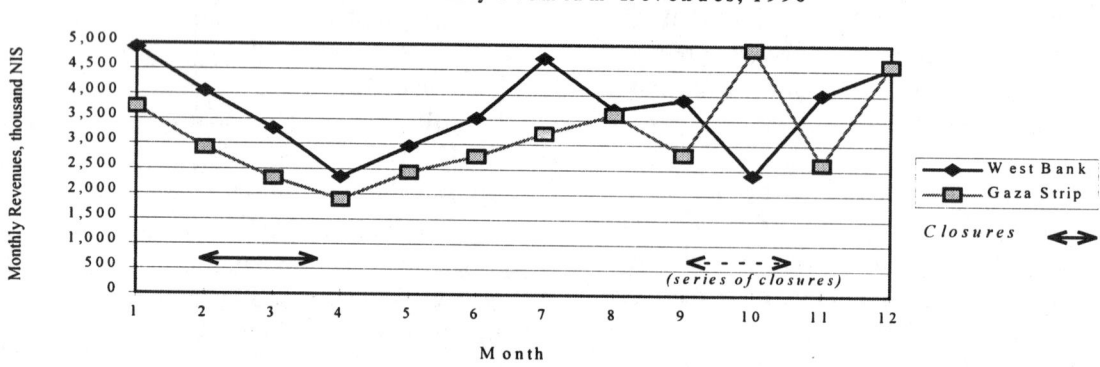

Source: Health Insurance Department, Ministry of Health 1997.

- The massive contraction of employment opportunities in Israel from 116,000 workers in 1992 to 28,000 workers in 1996 was totally unforeseen.

- It is estimated that between 1993 and 1996, border closures resulted in the loss of US$2.8 billion dollars which is equivalent to about 70 percent of annual GNP.

- The flow of external assistance to WBG has been much slower than initially expected. About US$1.3 billion of the pledged US$3.4 billion aid packet (to cover activities between 1994-1998) had been disbursed by the end of 1996.[3]

reflected in individual incomes. About half a million people live in poverty.[6] Poverty levels are higher in Gaza Strip, where about 40 percent of the population is estimated to be below the poverty line, compared to the West Bank where 10 percent is below the poverty line.

Consequently, the present bleak economic and political outlook is very different from the optimistic expectations at the signing of the Oslo Peace Accord. The severe disruptions to the economy have direct implications for the financial sustainability and the efficiency of the Palestinian health system. Health sector investment plans

---

[3] Forty four percent of health aid had been disbursed by the end of 1996.

[4] Unemployment rate includes individuals who are totally or temporarily unemployed.

[5] World Bank staff estimates.

[6] Poverty line is defined at $650 per capita per year.

Table 1: Selected Health and Social Indicators for the WBG and Selected Middle Eastern Countries (most recent estimates from 1993 to 1996)

	West Bank and Gaza	Jordan	Egypt	Lebanon	Tunisia	Turkey	Lower Middle Income Economies	Israel
GNP per Capita in US$	1,710	1,510	790	2,660	1,820	2,780	1,090	15,920
Population (million)	2.3	4.2	57.8	4.0	9.0	61.1	-	5.5
Infant Mortality Rate (per 1,000 live births)	28	34	57	32	40	49	60	8
Maternal Mortality Ratio (per 100,000 live births)	70	45	170	300	139	183	-	7
Total Fertility Rate	6.1	4.6	3.5	2.9	3.0	2.7	3.1	2.4
Adult Literacy Rate (percent)	84	87	51	92	67	82	-	95
Per Capita Health Expenditure in US$	122	118	38	124	105	99	-	1,114

Sources: Palestinian Central Bureau of Statistics 1996; Ministry of Health 1996; Health Nutrition and Population Sector Strategy, World Development Report, Hashemite Kingdom of Jordan Health Sector Study, the World Bank, 1997; The State of the World's Children, UNICEF, 1998.

prepared in 1994 were designed to achieve a rapid expansion of the health system[7] under the assumption of a relatively stable economic growth.[8] Many of these investments in the new health facilities are about to come on stream at a time when resources to operate these new facilities are declining. Figure 1 illustrates the impact of closures on the flow of revenues from health insurance premiums. The border closures also result in unexpected disruptions to movement and communications between Gaza Strip, the West Bank and East Jerusalem thus placing challenges not just on financing but on the flow of patients, staff, drugs, and supplies between these areas.[9] Responsibility for public health services in Gaza and Jericho was taken over by the Palestinian MOH in May 1994, while responsibility for the rest of the West Bank was transferred in December 1994. In spite of the enormity of problems facing it, the newly formed Palestinian MOH quickly succeeded in organizing an effective bureaucracy to administer and manage facilities transferred to it by the Israeli Civil Administration. At the same time the MOH began to assert its authority in the sector and define a sustainable long term strategy for the sector. The MOH needs to strengthen its strategic role and the present health system may be heading towards financial difficulties[10]. There is a risk that impressive gains already achieved as shown in major health indicators (Table 1) may not be sustainable.[11] The development of a long term health strategy is also hindered by both

---

[7] To compensate for previous presumed underinvestment prior to the Oslo Peace Accord.

[8] National Health Plan, 1994.

[9] The last internal border closure in September 1997 directly resulted in the documented deaths of at least 2 individuals and 4 births at Israeli checkpoints in the West Bank (MOH). Essential drugs and supplies in this period were distributed by international UN staff (MOH and UNRWA).

[10] Because of the recurrent implications of infrastructure investment and deteriorating macroeconomic environment.

[11] Economic recession in Latin America is estimated to have been responsible for 12,000 additional deaths in 1983, or 2 percent of all infant deaths in the region that year.

short term[12] and longer term political uncertainty.[13]

DEMOGRAPHIC AND HEATH STATUS

Compared to other economies at similar level of economic development, the Palestinian population is fairly well educated and overall health status is relatively good (Table 1). There are significant regional differences in socio-economic status and health status between the West Bank and Gaza Strip (Table 2). There are also large differences between the WBG and neighboring Israel.

Table 2: Regional Variation: Selected Health and Socio-economic Indicators (1996)

	West Bank	Gaza Strip
GNP per Capita (US$)	2,359	1,199
Infant Mortality Rate (per 1,000 live births)	25	32
Total Fertility Rate	6.9	7.4
Annual Population Growth (percent)	3.5	4.2
Adult Literacy Rate (percent)	90	76
Annual Household Health Expenditure (US$ per capita)	66	39

Source: Palestinian Bureau of Statistics 1996; World Bank staff estimates.

The epidemiological transition is underway and the leading causes of adult death are cardiovascular diseases (about 27 percent of adult deaths) and cancers (about 10 percent of adult deaths). On the other hand, diseases of poverty are still prevalent and respiratory infections and diarrheal diseases remain important causes of child mortality and morbidity. The latter conditions are due, to a large extent, to widespread poor sanitary (only 35 percent of households are connected to sewage networks) and environmental conditions. However, successful immunization programs (94 percent coverage) have been instrumental in controlling vaccine-preventable childhood diseases. Preventable accidents such as road traffic accidents and burns are important causes of childhood mortality and account for over a quarter of deaths in children between the ages of one and five.

Most of the population growth is due to natural population growth and the WBG has one of the highest fertility rates in the region (Table 1). Maternal mortality ratio is estimated at about 70 per 100,000 live births, which is significantly lower than several other lower middle income economies in MENA. While certain reproductive health services are well utilized (e.g. 93 percent of deliveries are attended by trained personnel), other services such as postnatal care and family planning are much less utilized (only 20 percent of women have postnatal checkups).

---

[12] Political and economic uncertainty after each violent incident results in a refocusing on short term issues such as provision of emergency services.

[13] The geographical separation between the West Bank and Gaza Strip remains a significant challenges to the development of an integrated health system.

Table 3: Hospital Capacity and Utilization Pattern, 1996

	Percent of Total Acute Bed Capacity (percent)	Size of Hospital/ Clinic (beds)	Bed Occupancy Rate (percent)	Average Length of Stay (days)
MOH Hospitals				
West Bank	35.0	50 - 142	84	2.8
Gaza Strip	36.1	31 - 402	81	3.2
NGO Hospitals	22.5	10 - 88/ [a]	64/ [a]	3.1/ [a]
NGO Maternity Clinics	5.5	10 - 12	24	1.2
UNRWA Qalqilya Hospital	1.8	38	114	2.8

a. West Bank only
Source: Ministry of Health 1997, WHO 1996. See Appendix 10 for further details.

2.   HEALTH SERVICE DELIVERY SYSTEM

INFRASTRUCTURE

There are four major health service providers in the WBG: the MOH, United Nations Relief and Work Agency (UNRWA), non-governmental organizations (NGOs), and private for-profit providers. The MOH provides both primary and secondary health services and purchases tertiary services from private providers domestically and abroad. UNRWA provides free primary health services to all registered refugees (regardless of income) and contracts other providers to provide secondary and tertiary services. NGOs provide primary, secondary and tertiary health care[14]. Private for profit providers range in size; from general physicians to advanced hospitals with a wide range of diagnostic and curative services. There appears to be increasing involvement of the private sector in the delivery of tertiary care and diagnostic services[15]. On the other hand, the MOH is also expanding its services at both primary and referral levels[16]. Thus there is a need to coordinate activities (including defining roles) among

the various health subsystems to reduce duplication and wastage of resources.

The MOH provides health services through its 14 hospitals and 209 clinics. NGOs and the private sector run 10 hospitals and 208 clinics. UNRWA runs one hospital and 41 clinics. The average MOH hospital bed occupancy rate in 1996 was about 83 percent (which is about the accepted range of optimal utilization) compared to 64 percent in NGO hospitals (Table 3) [17]. Although further analysis will be required to evaluate the hospital utilization patterns in detail, available government statistics indicate that inpatient admission rates in 1996 were around 9 percent (compared to 3 percent in Egypt or 8 percent in Tunisia). This is a relatively high admission rate for a young population with less than 3 percent above 65 years of age. Given the limited bed supply (currently around 1.1 beds per 1,000 population), this large number of inpatient admissions appears to be accommodated through a high turnover rate and a relatively short average length of stay of around 3 days[18]. This would suggest that some admissions may be unnecessary or that patients are being discharged too soon.

The uneven utilization rates among hospitals in different sub-sectors could indicate significant potential for improved efficiency

---

[14] The distinction between private and NGO providers is ill-defined. It appears that several NGOs may be evolving into for-profit organizations.

[15] For example, a private company is planning to open a new 120 bed hospital in Ramallah within the next two years.

[16] The MOH priorities (presented in June 1997) include plans for 100 bed expansion in Ramallah for tertiary services including neurosurgery and cardiac surgery.

[17] Excluding psychiatric hospitals.

[18] Actually 1.3 beds per 1,000 population if overseas referrals are included.

in the system.[19] Many MOH hospitals are operating at or above capacity, and overcrowding appears to be a problem at some of these hospitals. Meanwhile, most NGO hospitals are operating below capacity, particularly small NGO maternity clinics which have an occupancy rate of 24 percent. Part of the low utilization rate at NGO hospitals may be related to financing difficulties as patients admitted to NGO hospitals are not covered by the government health insurance program (GHI). Expansion of insurance benefits to include the NGO hospitals could help to increase their utilization rates, and hence promote a more efficient use of available capacity.[20]

Forty percent of outpatient visits occur in MOH facilities compared to 31 percent in UNRWA facilities and 29 percent with private practitioners or NGO facilities. Each UNRWA doctor sees 101 patients per day compared to about 51 per day seen by an MOH doctor in Gaza Strip. This difference is partially explained by greater likelihood of repeated visits in UNRWA clinics which usually serve a defined community and the high ratio of administrative physicians (about a third of PHC physicians in Gaza Strip are involved in administration). The effect of the number of patients seen per doctor on quality of services should be explored.

There are plans to expand the government sector by 97 additional clinics by 2002.[21] Efficiency could be improved by decreasing government-NGO overlap and integrating NGO/private clinics within the planned multi-level PHC system.[22]

The MOH recently assigned the Palestine Red Crescent Society (PRCS) the responsibility to establish comprehensive ambulance services throughout the WBG. Currently PRCS has 31 ambulances at 8 branches and 4 sub-centers in the West Bank which are connected with centralized radio-communication system. PRCS is preparing to start activities in Gaza Strip soon. However, the challenges in organizing an effective and efficient ambulance service are formidable. Such challenges include the underdeveloped phone and communication system and complex logistic issues (as the majority of major intercity roads are under Israeli control).

Box 1: Medical School

The only Faculty of Medicine in the WBG was established in 1994 at Al-Quds University in the West Bank. The Faculty is expected to take a leading role to standardize medical education which meets local needs in the WBG. The University is supervised by the Ministry of Higher Education. Each annual class intake for the 7 year program consists of 40 students. Although about 40 percent of the students are from Gaza Strip, some of them cannot attend due to logistic difficulties in moving to the West Bank. Tuition is JD 45 per credit hour with 35 to 40 credit hours required annually. Funds are available for poor students. The university opened a school of public health in September 1997.

HUMAN RESOURCES

Two thirds of the 7,000 health personnel in the WBG are employed by the MOH. There are about 56 doctors per 100,000 people in the West Bank and 78 doctors per 100,000 people in Gaza Strip. These ratios are similar to the regional average.[23] Currently more than 2,000 medical doctors who graduated from over 600 different medical schools are working in the WBG. Because of the wide

---

[19] Utilization rates in this report is used as a reflection of efficiency as it was the single consistent data measurement available across providers. Further detailed analysis including length of stay by specialty and case-mix as described in appendix should be carried out.

[20] The MOH is already contracting selected services from the NGO and private sector.

[21] MOH Priorities, June 1997.

[22] National Health Plan 1994; MOH priorities list, June 1997.

---

[23] The average numbers of doctors per 100,000 people are: 80 in the Middle East and North African countries; 30 in the lower-middle income economies; and 250 in OECD countries.

variation in the educational background of doctors, standardization in the quality of care is a problem that should be addressed quickly (Box 1). The MOH has made significant efforts in upgrading health personnel's skills through various training programs.

The licensing framework for physicians is being unified. In the West Bank, doctors are registered (after passing a licensing examination) by the Jordanian Medical Association (JMA) and then licensed by the MOH. The JMA also plays a role in fee setting, malpractice complaints, and medical education. In the absence of an active medical association in Gaza Strip, the role of the JMA is being temporarily played - pending development of an active medical association - by the MOH.

Many public sector doctors[24] work in their own private practices after regular office hours. It is prohibited for both specialists and general practitioners to practice privately in the West Bank, and it is legal only for specialists in Gaza Strip. However, because of low wages in the public sector, the MOH does not enforce these regulations (Table 4). The dual employment in both public and private sector may result in conflict of interests.

There are 4 different educational levels of nursing professionals: staff nurses with 4 year baccalaureate degree (BSN) or 3 year diploma program; practical nurses; and midwives. Training for these professionals are carried out at the 3 MOH nursing schools, UNRWA's 2 nursing schools and 3 baccalaureate level courses at private universities. The MOH has taken steps to improve the quality of the nursing professionals in the WBG by upgrading training courses of practical nurses and midwives, abolishing the training of nursing aides and stopping the hiring of traditional

birth attendants (TBAs) in public health facilities. There is at present a shortage of staff nurses in the West Bank in contrast to Gaza Strip where 500 staff nurses are unemployed. However, the restriction of movement of personnel makes it difficult to encourage relocation. The MOH is planning to more than double the number of nurses but this plan should be reviewed in light of budgetary concerns, employment patterns and identified needs[25].

PHARMACEUTICALS

A major achievement of the MOH has been the good and regular availability of drugs and vaccines. Very few economies have been through a period of rapid transition and turmoil without experiencing severe drug shortages. However, widespread availability has been achieved at considerable financial cost and drug expenditure is the fastest growing component of MOH's recurrent budget (increased from 22 percent of total health expenditure in 1995 to projected expenditure in 1997 of 32 percent). In 1996, total costs of drugs and disposables were estimated to be about 1.9 percent of GDP. Households spend about US$168 per year on drugs, or about 50 percent of their total health budget. Expenditure on the top ten

Table 4: Human Resources in Health

	Physician: Nurse Ratio	Basic Monthly Wage of Physicians
Ministry of Health	2:1/[a]	$625
United Nations Relief and Work Agency for Palestine Refugees in the Near East	1:1.8	$921
Private	1:1.4	$1,000 - $1,200
Nongovernmental Organizations	1:1.3	$900 -$1,000

a. Ministry of Health 1997.

---

[24] UNRWA physicians are allowed to run private practices after duty hours, farther than 10 kilometers from the particular UNRWA facility where they work.

[25] National Health Plan, 1994.

Box 2: Private Pharmaceutical Companies

There are 8 pharmaceutical companies in the WBG, none of which are producing drugs at Good Manufacturing Standards level. They produce about 50 percent of total consumption. Plant utilization is low and cost of production is high (with the best operating at perhaps two to three times higher costs than comparable factories in other countries). Israeli restrictions on importation from abroad protects the domestic industry from price competition, but also results in higher prices in both the public and private sectors. The domestic industry produces many combination products (with two or more active ingredients) which are generally marketed for product differentiation as opposed to any additional therapeutic values.

---

induced demand may play a role in inducing drug over-consumption and the ratio of pharmacies to population are much higher than small relatively densely populated European countries (1:4,071 in the WBG compared to 1:15,000 in Denmark).

drugs are responsible for about 25 percent of total MOH annual drug expenditure. The major impediments to rational and cost-effective development of the pharmaceutical sector are the lack of a national drug policy and antiquated non-unified drug legislation.

Drug prices are very high in the private sector (Box 2). MOH is reasonably successful in securing prices for most drugs which are not much higher than average international prices. However, UNRWA's prices are consistently lower. The Israeli requirement that drugs be registered in Israel is a hindrance to the import of low-cost generics into WBG.

There is a trend towards limited drug lists and many NGOs and UNRWA use such lists. The MOH tenders for only about 600 different drugs under generic names and a national essential drug list is in draft form. In spite of such initiatives, there is widespread over-prescription and polypharmacy, particularly of antibiotics, injections and combination products. The absence of standard treatment protocols makes it difficult to monitor and control prescription practices. Doctors in private practice rely primarily on expensive branded products and the present drug law does not allow for generic substitution. Supplier

Table 5: Government Services for Insured and Uninsured Population

Population Group	Type of Services Covered
Personal Care for All Population (insured and uninsured)	• Antenatal and postnatal care • Preventive and curative care for all children under the age of three (including immunization) • Hospital psychiatric services and community mental health programm
	• School health services: preventive and basic treatment during school hours in government schools • Public environmental health program
Benefits for Insured Population (50 percent of population)	• Primary curative care • Secondary care: hospitalization, including rehabilitation • Tertiary care, including overseas treatment or referrals to local private providers

Source: Ministry of health, 1997.

3. HEALTH FINANCING SYSTEM

The WBG devotes an unusually large share of its resources to the health sector. In 1995, health spending was estimated at about 9 percent of GDP[26], which is substantially more than most middle income countries (typically spend between 5 to 6 percent)[27] and several OECD countries (7 percent in UK, Denmark, and Japan).

MAJOR CHANGES IN HEALTH FINANCING

The health financing system that has evolved since the handover reflects both the features inherited from the Civil Administration as well as the aspects introduced by the newly established MOH. Prior to the handover, the notable features of the health financing system included: (a) a heavy reliance on external assistance[28] for a significant part of health financing (over 40 percent in 1991, including UNRWA), (b) relatively limited contributions from the Civil Administration, derived primarily from health insurance premiums accounting for less than a fifth of total health expenditure and only covering about a fifth of the Palestinian population), and (c) direct household expenditures that accounted for about 40 percent of the total health expenditures.

Since the handover, the following critical changes have occurred in the overall financing structure of the health system (Appendix 1 illustrates the present financing flows in the sector):

• Premium levels were reduced to encourage the expansion of coverage[29] (see Table 5 for services covered). This had the effect of lowering the total revenues from insurance premium

---

[26] World Bank data from latest available year (1990 - 1995).

[27] Schieber, G. and Maeda, A., World Bank, 1997.

[28] Including international NGOs.

[29] These new policies to encourage enrollment (e.g. by removing a waiting period) for the voluntary component of the social insurance scheme contributes to adverse selection.

despite the higher participation rate.[30] The shortfall has been increasingly covered by budgetary allocations from the government's general tax revenues.

- Donor contributions continue to be an important source of revenues for the health sector, but the main recipient of aid has shifted from the NGO sector (mainly providing basic services) to the MOH (80 percent of donor assistance directed to capital investment and capacity building).

- Overall international contributions to the health sector have probably declined, in real terms, in recent years (Table A 10.6, Appendix 10).

- UNRWA continues to finance basic health services for the refugee population. Its budget no longer keeps up with the rapid refugee population growth rate (over 4 percent).

- Private investors groups (particularly in urban areas of the West Bank) are entering the market primarily in tertiary care and modern diagnostic technology.

- The MOH appears to be replacing the purchase of overseas referral care with services provided by the emerging private sector.

ROLE OF PALESTINIAN AUTHORITY IN HEALTH FINANCING

In 1996, government spending accounted for about a third of total expenditure, direct out-of-pocket spending accounted for about 40 percent, NGOs about 7 percent and external donors (including UNRWA) about 24 percent (Table 6). The large external contributions partially explain the high level of health spending.

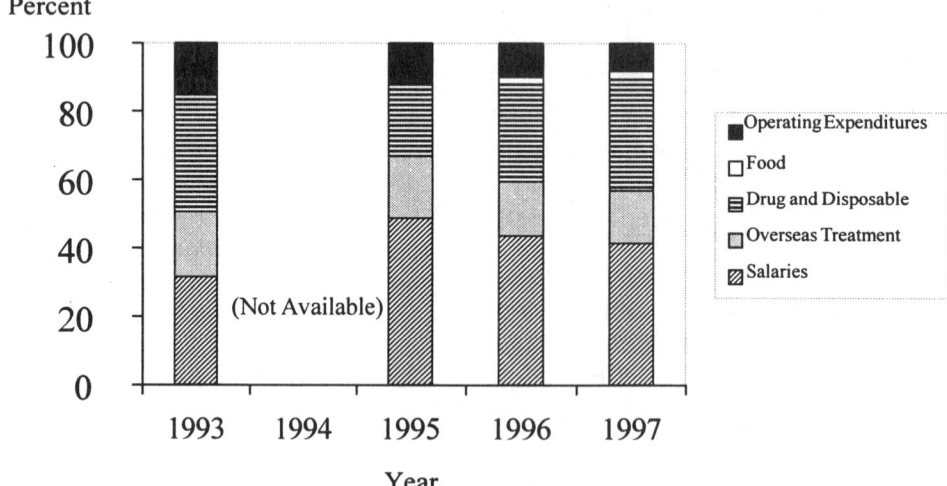

Figure 2: Ministry of Health Expenditure 1993-97

---

[30] Enrollment rates have grown fastest in categories - such as voluntary and group contracts - where it has being particularly difficult in reducing evasion of payments.

SOURCES OF FINANCING

Government health financing is derived from three sources: general taxation (about 60 percent), insurance premiums (25-30 percent) and copayments/fees (10-15 percent). Despite recent economic difficulties, government revenues have shown a strong growth over the period of 1995-97 due to the significant improvements in tax administration (see Table 7)[31]; and this reflected in a nearly 30 percent increase in health expenditure in 1996.

MANAGEMENT OF FINANCING

All revenues collected by MOH are transferred directly to the Ministry of Finance, and are reallocated to MOH through the annual budgetary process. Government providers are then financed through traditional administered line-item budgets, and are given little scope for financial management. The Health Insurance Department is an administrative division within the MOH, and does not function as an independent insurance agency. It functions primarily as a premium collection system for the MOH, and has an extremely limited role in the design of benefits packages and contracting of services. The MOH contracts services from overseas providers and a limited number of private providers which are usually negotiated on a case-by-case basis through the medical referral committees of the MOH. The MOH does not have a provider payment system that allows performance-based remuneration of providers.[32]

USES OF FINANCING

Figure 2 illustrates the recurrent expenditure pattern between 1993 and 1997. The very rapid growth in drug expenditure and the decline in the relative share of expenditure of salaries are major sources of concern. As discussed above, rationalization of drug use requires urgent attention. MOH salary increases have been held down for several

Table 6: National Health Expenditures in the West Bank and Gaza, 1991-97
(US$ millions, unless otherwise indicated)

	1991	1995	1996	1997 *(projected)*
Health Expenditure as Percent of GDP[/a]	8~9	8.6	8.6	Not Available
Real Per Capita Health Expenditure (US$)	$120~30	$125	$122	$111
Total Health Expenditure[/b]	224	276	~278 (100 %)	~263
Government Health Insurance	42	24	22 (8 %)	27[/c]
General Revenues	-	45	67 (24 %)	61
UNRWA	13	29	23 (8 %)	30
Donors	77[/d]	33	44 (16 %)	31
NGOs	-	37	~20[/e] (7 %)	~10[e]
Private[/f]	91	108	102 (37 %)	105

a. Includes capital expenditures, except for 1991.
b. Includes contributions from both international donors and NGOs.
c. Private expenditure includes household expenditure on health care, MOH copayments and private capital investments, but excludes household payments for government insurance premium.
d. World Bank staff estimates.
e. GDP, World Bank / IMF estimates.
f. Based on revenues in the first half of the financial year.
Sources: The World Bank, "Developing the Occupied Territories," Vol. 6, 1993; Barghouti and Lennock, 1997; and World Bank staff estimates. See Appendix 10 for details.

---

[31] Zavadjil, M. et al, "Recent Economic Developments: Prospects and Progress in Institution Building in the WBG; IMF, 1997.

[32] Individual publicly employed health providers are salaried.

years, and are fueling considerable dissatisfaction among MOH staff.[33] Any further deterioration in wage rates could have serious consequences on quality of care and may lead to labor unrest.[34]

Although the MOH already experiences serious constraints in available resources, measures needed for rationalization of resources and cost containment appear to be lagging behind. According to the latest current public investment plan, the MOH sector plans to expand its hospital capacity by 60 percent and its primary health care clinics by 20 percent by the year 2002.[35] This could imply US$50 million in annual recurrent costs in 2002 (at constant 1997 prices). This translates to an increase in budget of 11 percent per year in real terms in the next five years just to cover the additional recurrent cost of the expanded services (see Appendix 2, Table A 2.1 for details). This does not take into account the planned 10 percent increase in bed capacity in the private for profit sector. To cover the recurrent cost of the additional investment without increasing general revenue allocation, the GHI enrollment rate would need to increase by about 15 percent per year over the next five years at twice the present household contribution rate of US$130 per household (at constant 1997 price).

The proximity of Israel, with a per capita income almost ten times that of the WBG, has raised expectations on the part of the Palestinian population for a level of medical care and technology which might be difficult to sustain at their present income levels.[36] For example, the number of Magnetic Resonance Imagers (MRIs) per million population in the West Bank (1.6) already exceeds that of several richer economies

such as UK (1.4) and Canada (1.0). In addition to associated high maintenance and operating costs of such equipment, supplier-induced demand could result in rising health costs.

The MOH has initiated measures that begin to address its cost concerns (see Appendix 10 for further details). For example, the MOH is reducing reliance on costly overseas referral (accounted for 16 percent of MOH expenditure in 1996) for tertiary cases that cannot be treated within the WBG. In 1997 it is expected there will be zero growth in expenditure for such treatment due to a decreasing number of referrals to Israel (average cost of per case declined by about 50 percent). Cost pressures will be further exacerbated by the expected rise in demand for health services due to expansion of health insurance coverage, rapid population growth rate and the effects of epidemiological transition[37].

4. ACCESS AND EQUITY OF HEALTH SERVICES

Most of the Palestinian population have reasonable physical access to health care. According to a recent survey, more than 90 percent of the households in the West Bank and all the households in Gaza Strip have access to public and private clinics within 5 kilometers. Forty five percent of households in the West Bank and 74 percent of households in Gaza Strip have access to hospitals within 5 kilometers[38].

---

[33] A survey of MOH hospital staff indicated that a salary raise was one of the top two suggested administrative items that could result in improved quality.

[34] The legislative council recently approved a salary increase of about US$60 per month for doctors.

[35] Ministry of Health Priorities, June 1997.

[36] The Israeli health expenditure was around 7 percent of GDP in fiscal year 1990/91 (Chernichovsky and Chinitz, 1995). If we project the same percentage of health to GDP rate to 1995, it would amount to US$1,114 per capita expenditure on health, which is around nine times the per capita health expenditure in the WBG. Israel also enacted the National Health Insurance bill only in 1994, and is in the process of undergoing a major health sector reform to improve efficiency and contain costs.

[37] Likely to raise the per capita utilization of health services (moral hazard).

[38] Palestinian Household Survey, Palestinian Central Bureau of Statistics 1996.

Over a third of households are covered by the GHI. For insured households, the level of government subsidy in Gaza Strip (which has lower income levels, higher poverty levels and lower private per capita spending) is higher (Table 8). On the other hand, half of households have to bear the full cost of health care. Many of these households could probably afford to pay premiums, but are probably healthier and prefer to save on premium payments until they are ill. The relative ease with which one could join the GHI scheme probably encourages this behavior. Anecdotal evidence[39] suggests that certain groups, e.g. non-refugee poor are facing greater financial difficulties in accessing health care.[40] However, on the whole poor households spend less as a proportion of their total household expenditure on medical care when compared to other income categories (Table 8).

Table 7: Total Government Revenues and Health Expenditure, 1995-97

(US$ millions)

	1995	1996	1997 (projected)
Government Revenues	425	670	814
Total budget Allocation to Ministry of Health	69	89	88
General Revenues	45	67	61
Health Insurance Premium	24	22	27
Ministry of Health Budget (including insurance) as Percent of Total Government Revenues	16	13	11

Sources: IMF, 1997; Ministry of Health 1997.

Table 8: Percentage of household expenditure spent on medical care and estimated level of hospitalization subsidy per insured household

	Percent Household Expenditure (percent)	Hospitalization Subsidy per Insured Household (US$)
West Bank and Gaza	3.5	138
West Bank	3.7	113
Gaza Strip	2.8	179
Level of Living:		No Information
Worse-off	3.1	No Information
Middle	3.5	No Information
Well-off	3.8	No Information

Source: Palestinian Bureau of Statistics, World Bank staff estimates. See Appendix 10.

To improve financial access to health services, the MOH will need to expand coverage to currently uninsured population while ensuring that contributions are made according to ability to pay. There are certain aspects of the existing insurance system which are likely to present major obstacles to expanding coverage, maintaining solidarity and protecting access to care for the poor. They include: (a) the relatively low ceiling on monthly insurance premium payments (NIS 75) which establishes a regressive system of revenue collection and limits the contributions from the well-to-do; and (b) the voluntary nature of participation in the social insurance system that allows the well-to-do and low risk population groups to "opt out" of the system, (c) the relatively high refugee population who are entitled to free health care from UNRWA and (d) recent economic and political trends (such as high unemployment, declining wages and large informal sector).

[39] Based on discussions with the World Food Program which, in collaboration with the Ministry of Social Affairs, run a food supplementation program for the poor.

[40] About 20 percent of GHI enrollees are social welfare recipients whose premiums are fully covered by the PA. However, the relative high costs of co-payments may hinder financial access to health care.

5. DEVELOPING A NEW STRATEGY FOR THE SECTOR

The MOH faces unique challenges in attempting to develop a coherent health strategy to deliver quality services efficiently, while ensuring its financial sustainability, in a non-contiguous geographical area embroiled in an extremely complex political situation. The recent economic downturn can only exacerbate this challenge. However, inaction is not a viable option as it would lead to one or both of the following undesirable outcomes:

- Across the board underfinancing of the public system, resulting in a decline in the quality of health services[41], labor unrest, public dissatisfaction and deterioration in public support for the system and declining willingness to pay for the services.

- Increasing inequity due to reduction in resources available for subsidies, and increasing segmentation of the system as the private sector increasingly focuses on those who have the ability to pay and thus opt out of the publicly funded system.

To achieve the goal of ensuring a viable sustainable health system, certain priority areas need to be addressed in the short to medium term.

SHORT TO MEDIUM TERM: GETTING THE SYSTEM ON TRACK IN DIFFICULT ECONOMIC CONDITIONS

Organization and Management

Defining role and functions of various health subsystems. At present, coordination among the MOH (Box 3), UNRWA (Box 4), NGOs (Box 5) and private providers could be improved. The role and functions of each of the subsystems should be clarified and harmonized to reduce duplication and wastage of resources (see Appendix 3 for present structure). The MOH needs to define and strengthen its role with respect to its regulatory, policy-setting and coordinating functions; and to redefine and reevaluate its financing and service delivery/provider functions. The present structure would need to be reorganized to effectively carry out redefined roles and functions.

To be more effective in its regulatory and policy-making functions, the MOH will need to improve its capacity to collect and analyze policy-relevant data (such as the flow of funds through the establishment of national health accounts) in all sectors not limited to the public sector, and to assess the effectiveness of the subsidies and redistributive mechanisms in terms of ensuring equitable access to health services.

Financing

Reevaluation of the public investment strategy. There is an urgent need to review the present public investment plan in terms of their affordability and sustainability, with greater attention to improving efficiency. (See Appendix 7 for sample terms of reference). As a start, the investment requirements should be based on a better understanding of expected demand and utilization of services rather than on a static standards of capacity (e.g. two beds per 1,000 population). Rapid technological changes[42] render this traditional mode of investment planning obsolete. An investment plan should include specification of standards on buildings and equipment; projections of throughputs and estimations of fixed and variable costs at different levels of utilization; and the impact of public investments on the rest of the health systems (private, NGO and UNRWA).

---

[41] An MOH survey of patients in August 1996, revealed that 80 percent of patients were satisfied with their professional care.

[42] Such as the increased use of outpatient surgery.

Defining a benefits package. Definition of a benefits package would help to identify the priority areas for public financing. The list of benefits covered by MOH/GHI (see Table 5) is too general to be effective as a means for rationalizing services. A more refined definition of benefits package could be developed, e.g. through negative lists (services excluded from public financing) or positive lists (services included in public financing).

Improving complementarity between government and private/NGO hospital services. Expanding the benefits covered under the GHI scheme to include NGO and private providers would have the advantage of making a more efficient use of available resources as well as increasing the choice of providers for the patients. However, prior to expanding such benefits the MOH/GHI needs to improve its capacity to monitor the

---

Box 3: Organizational Structure of Ministry of Health

The MOH, headed by the Minister, is based in Gaza City. The Deputy Ministry is based in the West Bank city of Nablus. Six departments including Public Relations and International Cooperation report directly to the Minister. Seven departments including Health Insurance report directly to the Deputy Minister. Due to logistic difficulties and differing legal heritage, 6 administrative units including Financial and Administrative Affairs, Planning and Development, and Hospital Administration are duplicated in the West Bank and Gaza Strip (see Appendix 8 for further details).

Hospital administration is delegated to hospital directors who report directly to the respective Director General of Hospital Administration. While the management of service delivery is delegated to the 6 administrative units, budget and policy-making decisions are highly centralized. Certain decisions, such as the level of health insurance premiums, require the approval of the Legislative Council. In 1996, the MOH employed 5,838 staff, of which about 32 percent were employed in the administrative positions.

Box 4: UNRWA's Role in Health Care Delivery

UNRWA was created in 1949 with a dual role: to fulfill the humanitarian needs of Palestinian refugees and to defend their legal rights. UNRWA has provided, for almost 50 years, relief and social services, basic education and health care to the Palestinian population.

UNRWA is facing major financial problems. The increased demand of a growing population, coupled with a dwindling budget supported mainly by voluntary contributions (90-95 percent of total budget) from international donors. These donors appear to have reduced their financial support to UNRWA, preferring instead to support the PA bilaterally. This resulted in a financial deficit in 1996, which may yet threaten the delivery of basic services to the refugees. The agency has countered recent financial difficulties by introducing austerity measures, utilizing reserves while attempting to improve the efficiency and effectiveness of services provided. Nevertheless, it is clear that unless significant financial resources are made available, a reduction in extent and quality of provided services will be unavoidable.

Even allowing for the logistic advantages of providing services to a clustered population, UNRWA strategy and approach to health delivery has been efficient and could provide a basis to the development of a sustainable Palestinian health system. With an annual per capita expenditure on health of US$18, in a cultural and epidemiological situation similar to that of non-refugees, certain aspects of the UNRWA system e.g. treatment protocols and material resources management could be easily adopted and adapted to the government sector. Because of the economic and political implications, it is unlikely that the PA will accept the taking over of UNRWA's responsibilities outside an agreed political settlement of the refugee issue. However, a de facto harmonization of policies and service delivery between the MOH and the Agency would create the basis for a more efficient, less fragmented and more effective health system.

Box: 5 NGO's Role in Health Care Delivery

NGOs, in the pre-Oslo period, played a major role in the delivery of public services, particularly in the health sector. World Bank data suggests that between US$140-215 million in external funding was received by NGOs in 1992, the peak year for external funding - a sum that declined to perhaps US$60 million per annum in 1995 (of which an estimated 60 percent funded health activities). The precipitated cut in the funding base for health NGOs came about as the result of two factors first: the reduction of Arab support at the wake of the Gulf War; and second, the switching by western donors of a considerable proportion of their health financing to the PA.

Faced with this loss of support, NGOs adapted in a variety of ways. A few attempted to introduce fees for service while others elected to be absorbed into the PA. The majority, however, cut back on services by closing rural clinics and/or by reducing the range and frequency of services offered. Lack of funds for operating budgets appears to be a major reason for declining rates of occupancy in NGO hospitals (other reasons include the current access restrictions to East Jerusalem facilities, the types of services provided and the lack of insurance coverage for NGO services). Despite the existence of an informal MOH-NGO forum in which issues of mutual concern are discussed, NGOs have tended to react to the funding crisis and the changed realities of governance in an adhoc manner. The vision underlying the operations of many NGOs - independence in a financially unconstrained environment - no longer corresponds to reality, and needs to be adjusted. It will require the PA to develop effective public/private partnerships.

Developing a more integrated and efficient health system would require greater willingness of both PA and NGOs to see each other as sectoral partners.

---

quality, efficiency and costs of the private and NGO hospitals (see Appendix 7). This will involve the development of an appropriate provider payment system[43] that will facilitate the contracting of services between GHI and the providers. In addition, a potential conflict of interests exists between the government doctors who also have part-time private practice in the NGO/private hospitals and clinics.

Improving the complementarity between the private insurance market and public financing. The government will need to be more active in regulating the growth of the private insurance market (see Appendix 10). As a start, MOH will need information on the existing private insurance market, and to identify areas where better complementarity could be achieved between the GHI and private insurance market.

Harmonizing MOH and UNRWA payment schemes. Given the financial difficulties UNRWA is facing and the expectation that MOH and UNRWA services may be unified in the long term. UNRWA may consider, which might be difficult given its regional mandate, gradually introducing a similar co-payment scheme to that of MOH.

Provision: Infrastructure and Service Delivery

Rationalization of tertiary care subsector. Because of the serious long-term cost implications of investments in the tertiary care subsector, special attention should be paid to developing a coherent investment strategy in this sector (closely related to the development of a public investment plan). Priority should be given to the introduction of the most medically effective (evidence-based medicine), most appropriate (in terms of health outcomes and epidemiological profile of the population) and most cost-effective interventions. Consolidation of specialties within single hospitals rather than in providing multiple specialties in several small hospitals should be considered[44]. This exercise should be closely linked to a review of available medical technology as well as strategies for overseas referrals. There is

---

[43] For example, it is well known that an unmanaged indemnity system based on a retrospective fee-for-service payment can lead to serious cost-escalation problems without necessarily leading to better health outcomes.

[44] To ensure that medical staff do take adequate procedures to maintain their skills. For example the American Heart Association recommends that regional specialty cardiac centers perform at least 200 open heart surgeries annually.

some urgency in undertaking this review, since a number of investment plans are already being implemented in both the private and public sectors. Once established, a restructuring of the tertiary sector would be costly as well as technically and politically extremely difficult to undertake.

The government has two main instruments for influencing the growth of tertiary care services in the private sector. The first is through direct regulation of capital investment and medical technology, e.g. through licensing or issuance of a certification of need. The second is through its role as the purchaser, and increasingly a provider of tertiary care services. MOH will need to evaluate its current practice of reimbursing tertiary care services, and develop appropriate payment systems.

New approaches to delivering primary health care. As an alternative to direct expansion of the government-run primary health care system, MOH could explore the option of purchasing primary care services from other NGO clinics and private practitioners (especially in underserved areas). Such a plan could provide a more flexible arrangement to meeting the needs of the population, make use of existing capacities in the other sectors, and improve the complementarity and coordination of primary care services among the different subsectors. One possible strategy would be to contract qualified private practitioners to operate out of the government PHC centers. Such a primary care system could provide a clearer delineation of the roles and responsibilities of the physician and, if properly designed, could circumvent the problems created by salaried public doctors engaging in private practice. Another advantage is that it will also give the government greater flexibility in the management of PHC services, while introducing better regulation of the private practitioners. The ongoing pilot program for Family Doctors could be expanded to pilot such strategies, perhaps from the newly

constructed primary care facilities. (See Appendix 7).

Strengthening the referral system. An effective referral system needs to be established. Primary health care services should be strengthened to relieve the crowding and overuse of hospital services[45]. There is considerable scope for redesigning the co-payment system to discourage the unnecessary use of hospital care and promote the appropriate use of primary care. In principle, patients must be referred from the primary care physician to access hospital and specialist services, but at the moment there are no financial penalties for patients who choose to skip this process, and many primary care patients enter the hospital system through the emergency unit. However, any changes in the co-payment system should be accompanied by concurrent adjustments and improvements in the primary care services (e.g. better quality of care and longer operating hours in the government primary care clinics).

Strengthening hospital management. Greater involvement of public hospital managers in the area of financial management and cost containment would be essential for achieving better performance in terms of efficiency and quality of services. The MOH is already initiating some steps in this direction but these activities should be given a much higher priority in view of the increasing financial constraints. This will be a first step toward the introduction of greater managerial autonomy, and perhaps alternative hospital payment systems based on financial incentives that promote efficiency. These efforts must be accompanied by concurrent strengthening of financing and management systems, and management capacity (senior ministerial staff and hospital directors) to ensure such efforts are successful.

Improving preventive care. Greater attention needs to be paid to prevent non-

---

[45] For example, by expanding specialty care available at primary care clinics.

communicable diseases which are now the commonest causes of adult deaths in the WBG. Risk factors for these diseases (such as smoking and diet in the case of cardiovascular disease) should be targets of IEC campaigns. The preventive approach is usually much more cost effective than treating patients of non-communicable diseases.[46] The MOH has established a health education department which has initiated health education programs in selected schools.[47] Additional preventive interventions which can be started in the immediate future include:

- nutrition education and counseling to prevent diabetes, hypertension, and cardiovascular diseases;
- anti-smoking campaign;
- dental health education;
- health education and public awareness campaign against domestic accidents such as burn and traffic accidents;
- confidential counseling and home visits for mental and psychological disorders;
- advocating and counseling for family planning, and counseling to prevent genetic diseases;
- health education and public awareness campaign on sanitation and personal hygiene.

Provision: Human Resources

The MOH has already made significant efforts to upgrade capacity of human resources in the health sector (e.g. establishing the Health Services Management Unit). The following suggestions are made to build upon such efforts.

Develop a sustainable human resource strategy. A medium to long term human

resource master plan, which prioritize national needs based on financial sustainability, needs to be developed (see Appendix 7) [48]. Existing human resources may need to be re-trained or relocated in order to improve efficiency[49]. This plan should take into account the present job market and the changing role of health professionals.[50] Such a plan must encompass the training of professionals in universities and colleges (including the new medical school) to avoid oversupply of highly skilled staff (such as seen in Eastern Europe etc.).

This plan should closely complement the National Health Plan being developed. Improved planning and training of the health work force will not automatically result in improved patient care unless these workers are provided with work conditions (includes salaries and non-financial remuneration) and supportive supervision that stimulates them to excel, motivates them to provide quality services, and gives them professional satisfaction. In the immediate future, some of the savings from the new drug policies could be applied towards increases in staff salaries and benefits, but such stop-gap measures will probably not suffice to deal with the problem of low wage rates. The government will need to undertake an in-depth review of the wage structure and staff deployment strategies to come up with viable solutions for the medium-term.

Improving quality and technical efficiency. Protocols and standards for medical procedures and interventions need to be established quickly and integrated into various training programs. This has already being initiated (diabetes protocol by Quality

---

[46] For people eating a "western diet", a 60 percent reduction in salt intake would reduce the risk of death from coronary heart disease at age 55 by 16 percent and from stroke by 23 percent. World Development Report, 1993. World Bank. 1993.

[47] Partially financed by several donors.

[48] Such a plan should not be used to promote rigid central planning at the facility level where increasing autonomy is being encouraged.

[49] Between the West Bank and Gaza Strip. However, the lack of free physical access between both areas is likely to impede such a plan.

[50] For example, several OECD countries are rethinking the role of dispensing pharmacists as the role of pharmacy technicians and advanced information technologies increase.

Improvement Program) and UNRWA has been using such protocols in the past. It is suggested that a gradual move to using identical protocols in MOH and UNRWA be commenced. Explicit job descriptions are required for each category of health

professionals to clarify roles and responsibilities of each individual. The MOH has already taken steps to improve the quality of its services by establishing QIP (Box 6) which should be continued.

It is suggested that a unified licensing system should be established for all health professionals both in the public and private sector in the medium term. Such a licensing system could be used to promote continuing education and to harmonize the level of professional competence of professionals from various training background. The MOH, in collaboration with professional associations[51], should be responsible for monitoring the quality and efficiency of services provided using consistent and transparent indicators.

Provision: Pharmaceuticals

Given international experience in pharmaceutical reform, there is significant scope in reducing resources allocated for the pharmaceutical subsector which could result in the savings of up to 30-40 percent of present drug expenditure (Appendix 4). Because of the many stakeholders and vested interests in the pharmaceutical sector, any major reform needs not only to be carefully planned but should be implemented incrementally. Major issues in the sector would need to be discussed among various stakeholders and detailed studies are a prerequisite. Major pharmaceutical reforms would need to be closely linked to reforms in financing and provider payments. However, there appears to be, at present, sufficient information for pharmaceutical reform to begin.

Box 6: Quality of Services

There is some evidence that the quality of health services as perceived by providers[1] and patients[2] is inadequate. It is however difficult to provide an objective assessment of the situation due to limited available information. Quality can be accessed in terms of structural input (e.g. infrastructure drugs, personnel), process (what is actually done for the patient through delivering health care), and outcomes (the end results of correct processes and structural inputs). The PA, with help from several donors, has focused on the improvement of structural inputs e.g. building new infrastructure and equipment[3]. However, such improvements alone cannot correct process shortcomings which require quite different actions. For example, the non availability of a thermometer is a structural deficiency whereas the use of non-sterile equipment is a process deficiency.

The MOH has initiated a pilot quality improvement program at several sites including Rafidia Hospital. This program has resulted in several process improvements such as 56 percent reduction in turn around time for urgent laboratory tests and 92 percent reduction in waiting time at outpatient clinics. Perhaps more important than the actual improvements is the development of a quality culture in the hospital.

---

[1] Half of staff surveyed in Rafidiah hospital indicated that improvement in medical practice e.g. infection control was the most important priority in improving quality of care.

[2] The most important clinical priority of patient surveyed in Shifa hospital was improving medical practice (over 75 percent of surveyed patients).

[3] Inputs such as renovation of infrastructure (15 percent of patients surveyed in Shifa hospital) and medical equipment (2 percent of patients and 8 percent of health personnel surveyed in Shifa hospital) appear to be less likely perceived to be inadequate.

---

[51] The MOH should promote and encourage the development of professional syndicates.

Immediate (within one year).

- Approve and implement the essential drugs list, starting in public primary health care facilities;
- Finalize and introduce standard treatment protocols at all levels of care;
- Take steps to have the Israeli requirements on registration of imported drugs lifted for products from GMP certified manufacturers supplying the MOH;
- Introduce stricter requirements for the establishment of private pharmacies and restrict student intake to schools of pharmacy and the closure of one school of pharmacy should also be considered[52];
- Computerized central drug store management is implemented and improved methods for estimation of drug requirements are introduced;
- Combination drugs are removed from the market.

Short to medium term. It is recommended that once the suggested immediate reforms are being implemented that the following recommendations should be considered:

- Essential drugs lists for secondary public health facilities are implemented and then progressively introduced into NGO primary care services and hospitals, and drug co-payments and pricing are reviewed in collaboration with other financial changes[53];
- The capacity of the pharmaceutical sector administration and infrastructure is strengthened through additional technical staff, managerial training and equipment[54];

---

[52] It might be difficult to implement in the West Bank, at present, given the continuos threat of limited accessibility during closures.

[53] Fixed pricing is a standard feature in most Western European countries.

[54] The Ramallah Central Medical Store is renovated and equipped and the Gaza Store's first floor is completed and the store equipped.

- GMP certifications are established, and a scheme for generic substitution is developed, tested and implemented.

LONGER TERM: ACHIEVING UNIVERSAL COVERAGE

In the longer term, there are certain key issues - such as financing and delivery arrangements - which would need to be addressed. Detailed analysis of these are beyond the scope of this report but these key issues will be mentioned briefly.

Universal Coverage

The government has several options with regard to developing a system towards universal coverage. Two possible options are briefly outlined below (see Appendix 5 for further details). In both options, private insurance could develop a supplementary role to the public financing system.

Integrated health system. This approach most closely parallels the present investment strategy of the government, since it will involve the expansion of the public delivery system under the MOH rather than through the expansion of the purchasing function of the MOH. In a modification of this model, the single payer system- expansion of services may be achieved through contracting of services from private providers[55].

Many countries with this form of health system are experimenting with greater autonomy at the facility level and greater separation between provider and purchaser functions. This model relies primarily on taxation to finance the health system. However, most middle income countries do not have a sufficiently large tax base to be able to finance a full basic package of health services from government budget alone.

---

[55] Such as in Canada and increasingly in the United Kingdom.

Social insurance model. This will involve the establishment of a separate social insurance agency, or a group of insurance agencies operating under a public mandate. A major portion of its revenues will be derived through insurance premiums, but the funds will also require subsidies through general revenues to equalize access for different subgroups within the population. This system has the advantage of clearly distinguishing the health insurance functions from the other government functions, and making the process of health financing more transparent to the public. However, it will also involve a major restructuring of the health financing system in order to establish an insurance agency or a sickness fund that is independent from the MOH.

One potential drawback of this system is that in many middle income countries an independent social insurance agency or sickness fund have shown a tendency to develop their own, separate health delivery system paralleling the system financed directly by the MOH. It could lead to further fragmentation of the financing and delivery system, and to duplication and wastage of resources as well as inequities in access to services.

There is no single "correct" path toward universal coverage. Palestinian policy makers will need to weigh out the potential drawbacks and advantages of each approach (based on further information as suggested in Appendix 7) and select the approach that is in keeping with the social and political values as well as economic capacities of the country.

Hospitals

The existence of many small hospitals and clinics (approx. 10-30 beds), particularly in the NGO sector raises questions about the efficiency of the delivery structure. However, given the present political situation and geographical accessibility, these issues probably cannot be addressed in great detail in the short term. Within the hospital subsystem, there are areas where significant efficiency gains might be made. For example, a consolidation of specialties within single hospitals rather than in providing multiple specialties in many hospitals, may result in some degree of economy in scale and scope, and better outcomes from complex medical procedures.

6. PUBLIC FINANCING PRIORITIES AND CONCLUSION

The government has given high priority to its health programs and has developed a list of priorities for the period 1997-2002 presented to the Health Sector Working Group in June 1997. Based on the information in this document and assumptions of recurrent cost, it has been estimated that implementation of this program would require about US$422 million (includes about US$151 million in recurrent costs) over the next five years (see Appendix 2 of further details). This program is not likely to be financially sustainable in the longer term.

To illustrate this, the report assesses the financial sustainability of such a program as a share of projected GDP and public expenditures. If it is assumed that all capital costs (US$271 million) are financed by donors, the annualized recurrent costs implications of such a program would amount to 25 percent of the annual MOH budget in 2002 (further details and assumptions are available in Appendix 9). This would mean that by 2002, 12 percent of the PA budget would be needed annually to finance just these additional operating costs (Appendix 9) and is not likely to be financially sustainable in the longer term (Table 9). It would also reduce resources available for salary increase and might reduce resources available for primary care (as most of the rise in recurrent expenditure would be in secondary and tertiary care - see Appendix 2).

However, if the MOH is able to improve the efficiency of the health sector as reflected in average occupancy rate of 80 percent, to increase average length of stay to 4 days and reduce admission rates to 8 percent, the number of new hospital beds required in 2002 (assuming population growth and epidemiology remains constant) will be 1,036 beds (Appendix 2, Table A 2.2). This will represent 179 less beds than the present

Table 9 : Implications of Planned Capital Investment Program on Ministry of Health Recurrent Health Expenditure

	1997	2002
Recurrent Expenditure/ ($ million)	0	48.8
As Percent of Ministry of Health Expenditure	0	35
Ministry of Health Expenditure as Percent of Palestinian Authority Expenditure		
Scenario I	8.6	12
Scenario II	8.6	11.4
Ministry of Health Expenditure as Percent of GDP		
Scenario I	2.7	3.6
Scenario II	2.7	3.4

Note : Scenario I represents a GDP growth rate negative or equal to zero ; Scenario II represents a growth rate ranging between 2-3.5 percent.
Source : Appendix 9: Recurrent Expenditure.

public hospital investment plan (if the EU hospital is included). If it is assumed that 210 beds are provided by the private sector (as planned), the number of additional public beds required would be 826. This would reduce the cost of the hospital investment plan by US$63 million (resulting in a reduction of recurrent costs by about US$32 million). These costs are an illustrative scenario and do not take into account beds in East Jerusalem. If beds in East Jerusalem were easily accessible and the private sector provides 210 beds, the cost of the proposed hospital investment plan will be reduced by US$85 million (resulting in a reduction of recurrent costs by about $43 million). While these costs do not take physical accessibility into account, it indicates there is room for greater efficiency in resource allocation (Appendix 2, Table A 2.7).

For example, implementation of the present public investment plan (assuming no changes in admission rates) may result in occupancy rates as low as 26 percent in Jericho or 44 percent in Nablus (see Appendix 2, Table A 2.8). Thus, it is suggested that a national master plan that takes into account financial sustainability, utilization of health facilities and present resources is drawn up before major capital investment decisions are made.

To a large extent, the proposed plan focuses on the infrastructure development - which in itself cannot guarantee the delivery of quality services. The PA has the unique opportunity to avoid the development of an unsustainable infrastructure seen elsewhere and should harness this opportunity.

It is suggested to improve the efficiency and quality of health services, greater emphasis needs to be placed on the development of processes delivered by capable staff to deliver health services to the Palestinian people. The present economic and political challenges, only make this task more pressing.

Table 10: Implications of Suggested Capital Investment Program on Recurrent Health Expenditure

	1997	2002
Recurrent Expenditure ($ million)	0	40.2
As percent of Ministry of Health Expenditure	0	28
Ministry of Health Expenditure as Percent of Palestinian Authority Expenditure		
Scenario I	8.6	11.4
Scenario II	8.6	11.0
Ministry of Health Expenditure as Percent of GDP		
Scenario I	2.7	3.4
Scenario II	2.7	3.3

Note : Scenario I represents a GDP growth rate negative or equal to zero ; Scenario II represents a growth rate ranging between 2-3.5 percent.
Source : Appendix 9: Recurrent Expenditure.

The donors can help in two main ways to assist the Palestinians in achieving their health goals. They can: (a) support capacity building and training in management, policy-formulation and research, service delivery and information management that would result in the development of sustainable local institutions, and (b) provide financial support for investment program that supports the development of an effective and efficient health system. This may require a reassessment of present capital investment

plans[56] that may be detrimental to the long term financial sustainability of the health system. An important role for the PA, is to ensure adequate donor coordination to prevent overlapping donor financed projects and/or projects that might not be institutionally or financially sustainable by the PA in the longer term[57].

The World Bank and WHO have been partners with the PA and are prepared to continue to assist in the development of an effective and efficient health system for the Palestinian people. Other donors such as the Italian Cooperation (the Health Shepherd), the Japanese and the European Union have played major roles in the health sector. They and other interested donors would obviously be key players in implementing an investment program that supports the development of such a health system. It has to be recognized that the Palestinian health sector is not static, and the MOH has already started implementing several of the recommendations included in this report during the course of its preparation.

This report does not intend to be the final word on health strategy. Instead, it attempts to provide a focal point to continue the on-going dialogue on the future of the sector. It is suggested that this report be reviewed and discussed by various Palestinian constituencies and the donor community to bring the dream - of improving the health status of all Palestinians - closer.

---

[56] In 1996, the donors spent about US$43 million of which 62 percent went to capital investment

[57] The presence of an active health sector working group in the WBG is an initial step in this direction.

Appendix 1: FLOW OF FUNDS

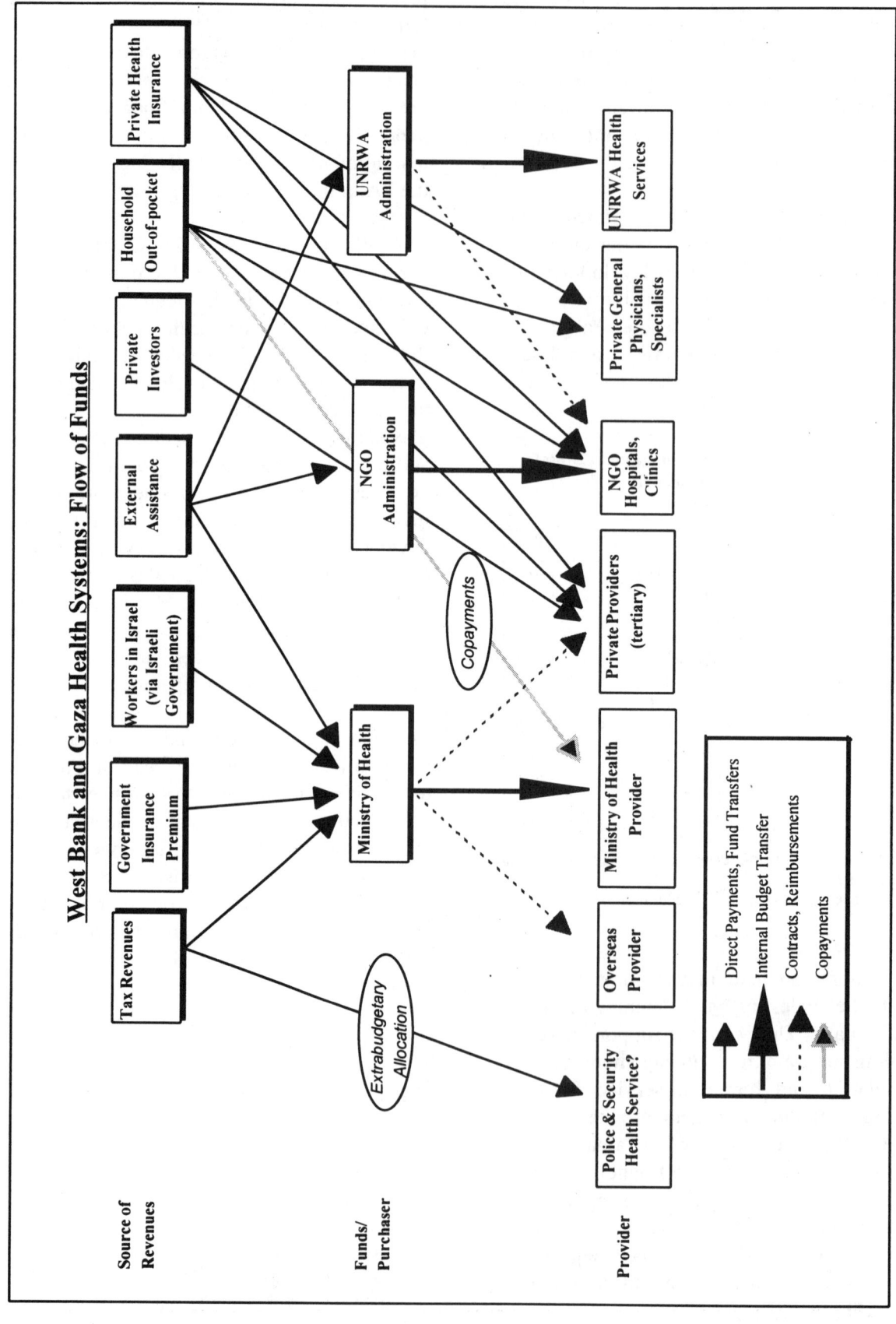

West Bank and Gaza Health Systems: Flow of Funds

Appendix 2: MINISTRY OF HEALTH PRIORITIES AND RECURRENT COST IMPLICATIONS
Table A 2.1: West Bank and Gaza Strip Ministry of Health Priorities, June 1997

Description of Investments	Number New Beds	New Beds, Facility	Upgrading	Rehabilitation Renovation	Equip-ment	Total
			US$ millions			
Tulkarem						
Tulkarem Hospital						
Phase I						
Emergency department, supply, kitchen, dining, laundry			2.0			
Blood bank, lab, X-ray, gynecology, physiotherapy, cardiac unit			2.4			
Phase II						
Staff residence, administration, pharmacy, ICCU, pediatric department			3.7			
Qalqilya						
Qalqilya Community Hospital	100	13.0				
Doora Community Hospital	50	5.0				
Yatta Community Hospital	50	3.0				
Beit Jalla						
Phase I						
Construction CSSD, linen store, workshops, OPD clinic			2.5			
Equipment					1.0	
Phase II						
Cardiac unit, X-ray, blood bank, administration, new beds	25	1.8				
Nablus						
Rafidiya Hospital						
Imaging Dept.			0.8			
Surgery Dept. 25 beds	25	1.5				
New Nablus Hospital (MCH)						
Phase I 120 beds	120	25.0				
Phase II 120 beds	120	15.0				
Jericho						
New Jericho Hospital, 70 beds	70	19.0				
Bethlehem						
Phase I						
Bethlehem Psychiatric Hospital chronic patient building			2.3			
Phase II						
Rehabilitation facility/building				3.2		
Jenin						
Jenin Hospital						
Phase I						
Emergency, Op theatre, X-ray, machinery/energy etc			4.5			
Phase II						
Construction of additional floor, adds 30 beds	30	5.0				
Hebron - EHRP/Saudi?						
Phase I						
Construction of 2 floors, pharmacy, machinery, dining etc.			7.0			
Phase II						
Expansion to 50 beds	50	3.0				
Ramallah						
Existing Hospital Building						
Renovation of medical dept and heart catheterization lab				2.4		
Angiography machine					1.4	
Construction (500sq.m.) new floor for ICCU, etc				1.1		
Construction of new floor (500sq.m.) for pediatric				1.1		
New Building						
Construction (2900sq.m.) emergency, day care etc			3.5			
Equipment for emergency, day care					1.5	
Expansion for neurosurgery, cardiac,orthop. ENT	100	10.0				
West Bank Subtotal	740	101.3	26.4	4.6	3.9	136.2
Gaza						
Shifa Hospital new building 8 floors						
Phase I - first three floors			7.3			
Phase II next five floors			5.1			
Phase III - equipment, furniture					3.7	
Shifa hospital - other upgrades & rehab			1.81	0.02		
Shifa hospital specialized surgery building, ne beds						
Phase I 60 beds, cardio, surgical, catheteriz., ENT	60	7.5				
Phase II - 70 beds: urosurgery, pediatric, neuro, plastic	70	5.2				
Equipment					4.8	
CT Scanner, Shifa hospital					1.3	
Children's Hospital						
Admin, storage, neonatal ICU, library, water tank			1.32			
Khan Younis						
Naser hospital						
Construction of 3 story building			1.6			
Equipment					0.6	
ICU, day care center, emergency, 37 beds	37	0.5				
Old Khan Younis Hospital - reconstruction				1.0		
Ophthalmic Hospital - OPD clinic, administration, hostel			1.0			
Middle Area						
Community Hospital (Dier El-Balah? EHRP/Saudi)	50	3.0				
Gaza Strip Subtotal	217	16.2	18.1	1.02	10.40	45.7
Other Equipment for West Bank & Gaza					33.2	
West Bank and Gaza Strip Total	957	117.5	44.52	5.62	47.5	215.2

Note : Cost of pyschiatric hospital has been not been
included in the total.

* 258 beds of the EU hospital under construction have not been included in the total
Source: Ministry of Health, 1997.

Table A2.3: Recommended Annual Investment for Hospital Sector, Including East Jerusalem

<u>Assumptions</u>:

Population in 1996	2,349,019	
Number of beds in 1996	2,640	
Population growth rate	4%	
Admissions	8%	
Average length of stay	4	days
Hospital occupancy	80%	
Bed replacement for new hospital	20	years
Bed replacement for old hospital	60	years
Investment cost/sqm (option 1)	$1,000	
Investment cost/sqm (option II)	$1,350	
Area required/bed	50	sqm

Year	1997	1998	1999	2000	2001	2002	Cumulative
Population (4 percent growth rate)	2,442,979.8	2,533,370	2,627,104.7	2,724,307.6	2,825,107	2,929,635.9	
Number of Admissions	195,438	202,670	210,168	217,945	226,009	234,371	
Number of Bed Days	781,754	810,678	840,674	871,778	904,034	937,483	
Beds Required (80 percent occupancy)	2,677	2,776	2,879	2,986	3,096	3,211	
Old Beds to be Replaced	45	46	48	50	52	54	294
New Beds Required	37	99	103	107	110	115	571
Total Beds to Construct	82	145	151	156	162	168	864
Investment Costs							
Option I	4,092,936	7,266,470	7,535,330	7,814,137	8,103,260	8,403,081	43,215,214
Option II	5,525,464.1	9,809,735	10,172,695	10,549,085	10,939,401	11,344,159	58,340,539
Recurrent Costs							
Option I 20 Percent	0	818,587	2,271,881	3,778,947	5,341,775	6,962,427	19,173,617
Option I 25 Percent	0	1,023,234	2,907,066	4,790,899	6,677,218	8,703,033	24,235,881
Option I 30 Percent	0	1,227,881	5,749,078	5,749,079	8,012,662	10,443,640	29,083,057

Note: Population estimates have been calculated assuming that approximately 20% of the E. Jerusalem population utilizes East Jerusalem hospitals area for construction of new hospital beds is 30 sqm in an existing hospital and 50 sqm in new hospitals. We took the higher figure of 50 sqm for our calculations.
Source: World Bank Staff Calculations.

Table A2.4: Recommended Annual Investment for Hospital Sector, Excluding East Jerusalem

Assumptions:

Population in 1996	2,280,000
Number of beds in 1996	2,080
Population growth rate	4%
Admissions	8%
Average length of stay	4 days
Hospital occupancy	80%
Bed replacement for new hospital	20 years
Bed replacement for old hospital	60 years
Investment cost/sqm (option 1)	$1,000
Investment cost/sqm (option II)	$1,350
Area required/ bed	50 sqm

Year	1997	1998	1999	2000	2001	2002	Cumulative
Population (4 percent growth rate)	2,371,200	2,458,934.4	2,549,915	2,644,261.8	2,742,099.5	2,843,557.2	
Number of Admissions	189,696	196,715	203,993	211,541	219,368	227,485	
Number of Bed Days	758,784	786,859	815,973	846,164	877,472	909,938	
Beds Required (80 percent occupancy)	2,599	2,695	2,794	2,898	3,005	3,116	
Old Beds to be Replaced	43	45	47	48	50	52	285
New Beds Required	519	96	100	103	107	111	1,036
Total Beds to Construct	562	141	146	152	157	163	1,321
Investment Costs							
Option I	28,094,247	7,052,967	7,313,926	7,584,542	7,865,170	8,156,181	66,067,032
Option II	37,927,233	95,215,04.9	9,873,800.6	10,239,131	10,617,979	11,010,844	89,190,493
Recurrent Costs							
Option I 20 Percent	0	5,618,849	7,029,442	8,492,228	10,009,136	11,582,170	42,731,826
Option I 25 Percent	0	7,023,561	8,786,803	10,615,285	12,411,420	14,477,713	53,414,783
Option I 30 Percent	0	8,428,273	10,544,164	12,738,342	15,013,704	17,373,255	64,097,739

Note : Recommended area for construction of new hospital beds is 30 sqm in an existing hospital and 50 sqm in new hospitals. We took the higher figure of 50 sqm for our calculations.

Number of beds required in 1997 is the difference between existing number of beds in the WBG (2,080) and those required to match population needs in 1997 at 8% admission rate, 80% occupancy and average length of stay of 4 days. Number of beds required for rest of the years is equivalent to old beds needing to be replaced every year and new beds to be constructed to meet the needs of the population as it grows.

Source: World Bank Staff Calculations.

Table A2.5: Total Recommended Investment 1997-2002,
Including East Jerusalem

West Bank and Gaza including European Union	1997	1998	1999	1998	2001	2002	Cumulative
Hospital Investment	23.60	23.60	23.60	23.60	23.60	23.60	**141.64**
Recurrent Cost 20 Percent	0	4.72	9.44	14.16	18.88	23.60	70.80
Recurrent Cost 25 Percent	0	5.90	11.80	17.70	23.60	29.50	88.50
Recurrent Cost 30 Percent	0	7.08	14.16	21.24	28.32	35.40	106.20
PHC Investment	11.1	8.5	8.5	6.9	4.2	4	**43.1**
Recurrent Cost 30 Percent	0	3.3	5.9	8.4	10.5	11.8	39.9
Recurrent Cost 40 Percent	0	4.44	7.84	11.24	14	15.68	53.2
Other Investment							
I. Ambulance Services	0.83	0.83	0.83	0.83	0.83	0.83	5.00
II. Buildings							
Public Health Laboratory	0.47	0.47	0.47	0.47	0.47	0.47	2.80
Laundry Building	0.04	0.04	0.04	0.04	0.04	0.04	0.25
Nursing School	0.25	0.25	0.25	0.25	0.25	0.25	1.50
Central Stores	0.42	0.42	0.42	0.42	0.42	0.42	2.50
Maintenance Workshop	0.04	0.04	0.04	0.04	0.04	0.04	0.25
Sub Total Buildings	1.22	1.22	1.22	1.22	1.22	1.22	7.30
Total Other Investments							12.30
Recurrent Cost of Other							
Ambulance 15 Percent	0	0.12	0.31	0.49	0.67	0.85	2.45
Miscellaneous Buildings 5 Percent	0	0.06	0.12	0.18	0.24	0.30	0.91
Total Investment Cost	36.75	34.15	34.15	32.55	29.85	29.65	197.04
Total Recurrent Cost	0.00	8.24	15.75	23.26	30.30	36.52	114.06

Note: All costs are in US$ million.

Hospital Investment includes construction cost of additional hospital beds needed by MOH [App. 2c, option I] plus costs of upgrading, rehabilitation and equipment as budgeted in MOH June Priorities, 1997 [App. 2a].

Recurrent cost calculated using hospital cost @ 20% of investment, PHC @ 30% and recurrent cost of other investments as their given rates. Rates for calculation of recurrent cost vary from 20 - 33% for hospitals and are higher for smaller facilities.

Source: M. Hopkinson and K. Kostermans, Building for Health Care, World Bank 1996.

Table A2.6: Total Recommended Investment 1997-2002,
Excluding East Jerusalem

West Bank and Gaza including European Union	1997	1998	1999	1998	2001	2002	Cumulative
Hospital Investment	27.27	27.27	27.27	27.27	27.27	27.27	**163.64**
Recurrent Cost 20 Percent	0	5.45	10.91	16.36	21.82	27.27	81.82
Recurrent Cost 25 Percent	0	6.85	13.64	20.46	27.27	34.09	102.28
Recurrent Cost 30 Percent	0	8.18	16.36	24.55	32.73	40.91	122.73
PHC Investment	11.1	8.5	8.5	6.9	4.2	4	43.1
Recurrent Cost 30 Percent	0	3.3	5.9	8.4	10.5	11.8	39.9
Recurrent Cost 40 Percent	0	4.44	7.84	11.24	14	15.68	53.2
Other Investment							
I. Ambulance Services	0.83	0.83	0.83	0.83	0.83	0.83	5.00
II. Buildings							
Public Health Laboratory	0.47	0.47	0.47	0.47	0.47	0.47	2.80
Laundry Building	0.04	0.04	0.04	0.04	0.04	0.04	0.25
Nursing School	0.25	0.25	0.25	0.25	0.25	0.25	1.50
Central Stores	0.42	0.42	0.42	0.42	0.42	0.42	2.50
Maintenance Workshop	0.04	0.04	0.04	0.04	0.04	0.04	0.25
Sub Total Buildings	1.22	1.22	1.22	1.22	1.22	1.22	7.30
Total Other Investments							**12.30**
Recurrent Cost of Other							
Ambulance 15 Percent	0	0.12	0.31	0.49	0.67	0.85	2.45
Miscellaneous Buildings 5 Percent	0	0.06	0.12	0.18	0.24	0.30	0.91
Total Investment Cost	40.42	37.82	37.82	36.22	33.32	33.32	**219.04**
Total Recurrent Cost	0.00	8.97	17.22	25.47	33.23	40.19	**125.08**

Note: All costs are in US$ million.

Hospital Investment includes construction cost of additional hospital beds needed by MOH [App. 2c, option I] plus costs of upgrading, rehabilitation and equipment as budgeted in MOH June Priorities, 1997 [App. 2a].

Recurrent cost calculated using hospital cost @ 20% of investment, PHC @ 30% and recurrent cost of other investments as their given rates. Rates for calculation of recurrent cost vary from 20 - 33% for hospitals and are higher for smaller facilities.

Source: M. Hopkinson and K. Kostermans, Building for Health Care, World Bank 1996.

Table A2.7: Summary of Possible Savings in Investment

Hospital Investment	Beds	Capital Cost (US$ million)	Cumulative Recurrent Cost (US$ million) - including operating cost of European Union hospital
1. Ministry of Health Investment Plan	957 258 1,215[a]	215 N. A	108[b]
2. Recommended Investment for Whole Sector Excluding East Jerusalem	1,036	163[c]	82
3. Savings on Ministry of Health Plan (subtracting item 2 from item 1)	179	52	26
4. Adjusting for Proposed Private Investment by Reducing 210 beds	826	152 .5	76
5. Total Adjusted Savings on Ministry of Health plan (subtracting item 4 from item 1)	389	62.5	32
6. Recommended Investment for Whole Sector Including East Jerusalem	571	141[c]	71
7. Savings on Ministry of Health Plan (subtracting item 6 from item 1)	644	74	37
8. Adjusting for Proposed Private Investment by Reducing 210 beds	361	130.5	65
9. Total Adjusted Savings on Ministry of Health Plan (subtracting item 8 from item 1)	854	84.5	43

Source: World Bank Staff Calculations.

a   957: Ministry of Health, 258: EU hospital.

b   Including operating cost of EU hospital.

c   Also includes cost of replacement beds, upgrading and equipment.

Table A2.8: Implication of Additional Beds on Occupancy
of Ministry of Health Hospitals by Region

Assumptions:

Estimates of additional beds taken from MOH Priorities, June 1997.

Admission rate of 1996 based on discharge data of the various MOH hospitals, May 1997.

Admission rate for 2002 is based on the 1996 rate with only incremental changes in patient population due to population growth rate of 3.7 percent.

Average length of hospital stay for 1996 by different regions, obtained from Annex 2 and kept constant for projections.

Region		Existing Beds 1996	Admissions 1996	Bed Days 1996	Occupancy 1996 (Percent)	Total Beds 2002	Admissions 2002	Bed Days 2002	Occupancy 2002 (percent)
Tulkarem		84	8,418	18,800	80	84	10,468	23,343.6	76
Qalaqilya		0				200			
Beit Jala		70	6,390	21,085	82	95	7,946	26,221.8	76
Jericho		50	3,133	9,001	49	120	3,896	11,181.5	26
Beit Lahem		-				-			
Jenin		55	12,435	23,667	118	85	15,464	30,928.0	100
Ramallah		142	11,601	43,301	83	242	13,912	51,474.4	58
Hebron		103	16,804	38,401	102	153	20,897	48,063.1	86
Nablus	[Al Watani]	86	7,340	21,867	69				
	[Rafidia]	138	16,573	41,678	83				
	Sub total	224	23,913	63,545	77	489	29,738	79,103.1	44
Gaza City		433	38,494	128,581	81	563	47,870	157,971.0	77
Khan Younis		318	34,575	97,126	84	355	42,997	120,391.6	93
Middle Area						50			

Note: Chronic care beds such as psychiatric beds have not been included.
Source: For number of beds : Annex 2

Appendix 3: STRUCTURE OF HEALTH SYSTEM

Table A3.1: Structure of the Health System: Entitlements, Financial Responsibilities and Principal Providers in the West Bank and Gaza, 1996

Type of Services	Entitlement /[a]	Direct Financial Responsibility (principal payers)	Principal Providers
All Population:			
Preventive Care, Including Early Child Care (0-3 years); Antenatal and Postnatal Care	All citizens/[a]	Government	Government, NGOs
Basic Curative Care	GHI holders (50 % of households)	Government (budget, GHI), households (fees)	Government, private, NGOs
Secondary and Tertiary Care	GHI holders, police and security forces	Government(budget, GHI), households (premium, co-payments or fees for service)/[b]	Government, NGO/ private, overseas providers
Rehabilitation	All citizens	Government, NGOs	NGO
Mental Health	All citizens	Government	Government/ NGOs
Dental	Selective services covered by government health service	Government, households (fees for service)	Government, private, NGO
Registered Refugee Population:/[c] Primary Care	Free care for refugees	UNRWA (external assistance)	UNRWA
Secondary Care	A limited number of cases approved for referral	UNRWA, households (cost-sharing)	Subcontracted hospitals (NGO, overseas), one UNRWA hospital

a. "Entitlement" refers to those services for which the citizens of the West Bank and Gaza are, in principle, guaranteed some level of public financing: it is not equivalent to actual access to services, since that depends on the actual availability of government services in the area.

b. Social welfare cases have health insurance premiums paid by the government.

c. As noted in the text, the refugee population also have access to all of the government services if they participate in the GHI plan.

Source: Ministry of Health, United Nations Relief and Work Agency for Palestine Refugees in the Near East.

Appendix 4: SAVINGS OF PHARMACEUTICAL REFORMS

Activity	Savings (percent)
Implement National Drug Policy and Legislation	5
Introduce Essential Drugs List at All Health Care Levels	5-10
Improve Ministry of Health Procurement	10
Implement Standard Treatment Protocols in Public Health Facilities	5-10
Introduce and Enforce Generic Substitution	5-10
Improve Storage and Distribution Management	5-10
Shift from Injections to Tablets and Capsules When Justified	2-5
Remove Inappropriate Drugs from the Market	3-5
Total Rationalization of Drug Sector	**30-40**

Source: World Bank Staff Calculations.

Appendix 5: DIFFERENT MODELS OF HEALTH FINANCING AND MANAGEMENT SYSTEMS

	Single Payer System	Integrated Health System	Social Insurance System
Examples	Canada - financed mainly by taxation with mainly private providers	UK / Scandinavian countries, Portugal - financed mainly by taxation with mainly public providers	Germany, France, Belgium - financed mainly by social insurance with mixed public and private providers Netherlands - financed by a mixture of social and private insurance with mainly private providers
Type of Public Purchasing Agency	Provincial, regional or local health authority	Ministry of Health, regional/local health authorities, municipalities	Sickness fund, social security agency
Main Source of Revenue	General tax revenues	General tax revenues	Payroll tax, employer and employee contributions
Typical Hospital Payment Systems	Contracts and other forms of provider payment system with autonomous providers	Direct administrative control with salaried personnel and budget transfers; increasingly, this system is being replaced by contracts with semi-autonomous public providers	Contracts, and other forms of prospective payment systems with autonomous providers (private and public)
Typical Physician Payment Systems	Fee-for-service with referrals required for specialist services	Salaried physicians; general practitioners, fundholding, fee-for-service with referrals required for specialist services	Fee-for-service, sometimes with balanced billing
Private Insurance	Mainly supplementary to public financing	Mainly supplementary to public financing	Mainly supplementary to social insurance; certain groups, e.g. the wealthy, are allowed to finance their health care services entirely from private insurance

Source: World Bank.

Appendix 6: ESTIMATED OF LEVELS OF SUBSIDIES

	West Bank (US$ thousands) Actual	Percent	Gaza Strip (US$ thousands) Estimation/1	Percent	WBG (US$ thousands) Estimation/1	Percent
MOH Health Expenditure						
Overseas Treatment	9,231	19	6,476	13	15,707	16
Hospital	21,953	45	22,659	45	44,612	45
Primary Care	11,073	23	11,429	23	22,502	23
Other	6,258	13	9,511	19	15,769	16
Total	48,515	100	50,075	100	98,590	100
Number of Insured Households	102,723		73,787		176,510	
Cost of Hospitalization per Household (US$) /2	295		386		333	
Contribution per Household	168		181		176	
Copayment per Household	14		26		19	
Subsidy per Household	113		179		138	
Subsidy as Percent of Premium Contribution	67		99		78	

1. For Gaza Strip, the distribution of expenditure between hospital and public health sectors was assumed to be the same as in the West Bank.
2. About 10 percent of hospitalization is assumed to be uninsured population. Therefore the total expenditure on hospital for the insured population was reduced by 10 percent.
Source: Ministry of Health, World Bank Staff Calculations.

Appendix 7: FOLLOW UP STUDIES ON HEALTH SECTOR IN THE WEST BANK AND GAZA

Exploring Options for Financing with Relevance to Macroeconomic Scenario

Sources of financing of health care in the country are currently fragmented and a more coherent strategy for revenue generation is needed. Attention needs to be given as to how will additional revenues be raised such that they are well tied to the overall macro-economic scenario.

i.   <u>Assessing flow of funds outside the health sector</u> : To come up with sources for financing, it would be extremely useful to explore the general flow of funds outside the health sector. The study should look at what taxes are raised and spent at both national and local levels; what flexibility is available in the current legal framework for raising taxes at local levels; how much flexibility there is in spending national budgets at the local level. The information can be helpful in designing both sources and use of health financing.

ii.   <u>Analyzing impact of different tax collection mechanisms</u> : Different options for tax collections can be studied and simple simulation models set up to look at the impact of different tax options such as payroll tax, earmarked taxes, VAT, general revenues, copayments or premiums etc. For example, is revenue generation tied to employment a good idea given the volatility of the labor market, will payroll tax only hurt economic growth by discouraging small businesses or is VAT a better option and feasible to implement.

Feasibility Study on the Expansion of the Government Health Insurance System

This study will evaluate the feasibility of alternative options for medium and long-term strategy for expanding the coverage of Government Health Insurance System towards the goal of universal coverage, and will include the evaluation of the private insurance market as part of the overall strategy. The study will involve field data collection, data analyses, and the presentation of various policy scenarios based on different options which will be used for future policy formulations and policy decisions by the Palestinian Authority. The study will offer recommendations on various options for changes in the design of the GHI to expand coverage and achieve adequate social protection, while maintaining financial solvency and promoting efficient delivery of services.

The study will comprise the following subcomponents:

i.   <u>Analysis of the determinants of demand for health insurance:</u> The 1996 household consumption and expenditure surveys collected by the Palestinian Central Statistical Bureau in 1996 provides valuable source of data on the characteristics of households with and without insurance, including income levels, household size and composition, geographical location and employment status. The 1996 data would be supplemented by sample surveys of households on their health status, utilization of health services, and income profile, including the impact of border closures on the household expenditures on medical care and insurance. These household data will provide critical information on the demand for insurance that are necessary for identifying major obstacles to expanding coverage, as well as estimating the effects on the GHI system of income fluctuations (border closures), changes in the premium levels, and other changes in the design of the insurance plan.

ii.   Social Welfare Cases: The effectiveness of the existing GHI system in providing adequate financial protection to the social welfare recipients will be analyzed under this subcomponent. Among the issues to be analyzed by this study will include a review of the affordability of the copayment system for the indigent population, and the adequacy of social welfare program in identifying households in need.

iii.   Flow of Funds Analysis of the GHI System: Revenue and Expenditure Patterns: At present the GHI system operates as a part of the government budget system and does not function as an independent fund. Consequently, it is difficult to follow the flow of funds from its source and its final use, and to evaluate the effectiveness of the system. This component of the study will analyze the financial data to determine the actual expenditures on major categories of benefits provided by the GHI system, evaluate the efficiency of fund use, and make recommendations on ways to improve efficiency and strengthen the financial management and accountability of the system. In addition, the study will make projections on the revenues and expenditures of the GHI system under a variety of policy scenarios.

iv.   Participation of the Employers and Corporations in the GHI: Eliciting a more active participation and contributions into the GHI system from the employers and corporations will be critical for future sustainability of the GHI funds. This component of the study will review the current involvement of the formal employment sector in providing health benefits to their employers and their relations to the labor laws, identify opportunities for promoting greater participation of the employer groups in the GHI scheme, and offer recommendations for the health insurance legislation with regard to the responsibilities of the employer.

v.   Role of the Private Insurance Market in Expanding Health Coverage: Private insurance will play an increasingly important role in the financing of health services in the WBG. The first part of the study will focus on collecting data on the extent and types of services covered by the private insurance companies, and identifying key issues and challenges facing the private insurance companies. The second part of the study will promote a dialogue between the government and private sector representatives to develop a policy framework for establishing an effective private insurance market within the context of expanding GHI system. Issues to be discussed will include: the complementarity of benefits financed by private insurance and GHI system, supplementary financing of GHI system through private insurance, and regulation of the private insurance market.

Promoting a Rational Investment Strategy for the Public and Private Hospital Sector - Facility and Equipment Planning

The present public investment plan does not take into account ongoing expansion in the non-public sub-sectors. Therefore it can result in greater inefficiency in terms of utilization of health facilities and will also be difficult to sustain financially. It is suggested that a national master plan that takes into account financial sustainability, utilization of facilities and present resources is drawn up before making major capital investment decisions.
For details see Appendix 7b.

Study on Improving the Quality and Efficiency of Hospital Services and Promoting Private / Public Complementarity

While the government is planning a major expansion in the public hospital system, relatively less attention has been focused on improving the efficiency of the public hospitals or making greater use of the existing NGO and private hospital capacity. This study will help to establish the necessary baseline data and provide training and technical assistance in the following areas:

i.   Strengthening management and quality of services in public hospitals: This component will expand upon the various studies and training in hospital cost analysis, financial management and quality improvement, and integrate these into a comprehensive hospital management training and evaluation program.   This will also include the establishment of financial management and cost accounting system, establishment of quality benchmarks and evaluation systems for various wards and departments, and comparative analysis of unit costs, expenditure and utilization patterns of each hospital.

ii.   Improving Complementarity of Services with Private Hospitals: At present only a few private hospitals receive reimbursements from the GHI system, and for only a very limited category of treatments and diagnoses.   Expanding the benefits covered by GHI to include services provided at private hospitals will be an important step in providing efficient services as well as offering greater choice of providers to the patients. This component of the study will gather information and identify the measures needed to support the expansion of GHI system to private hospital care. The study will help to collect data on the capacities, costs, utilization patterns and quality of services provided by various private and NGO hospitals. These data will form the basis for establishing appropriate tariffs and provider payment systems with the private providers.   In addition the study will support the government efforts in developing a clear regulatory and legal framework for the GHI system as it pertains to the rights and responsibilities in relation to any contractual arrangements with private entities. These steps are essential in strengthening the accountability of the public system, averting collusion and conflict of interest, and applying appropriate sanctions against fraudulent activities.

Improving the Efficiency of the Primary Health Care System

This study will focus on improving the efficiency and quality of the primary health care system to complement the major expansion in the government PHC system over the medium-term. The expansion in the PHC system will entail a substantial increase in the staffing to operate the system. However, the number of MOH staff and wage rates are not likely to increase sufficiently over the next five years to meet the proposed expansion of PHC services.   This study will assist the government in examining the feasibility of alternative approaches to expanding the PHC services through arrangements that make efficient use of existing resources while promoting quality and professional improvements. For this purpose, more data on the availability and qualifications of private physicians will be necessary. The activities to be supported by this study could include:

•   Survey of private practitioners in the WBG with respect to their numbers, qualifications, fees charged and number of visits by patients;
•   Review of private insurance payments for various categories of private physicians, including any group contracts;

- Testing the feasibility of contracting with private physicians to work in government PHC clinics, either on a full or part-time basis;
- Development of a prototype for physician payment system for the GHI system;
- Linking quality assurance and continuing education program for physicians with licensing and contractual arrangements with the GHI system;
- Strengthening of the referral system based on better training of primary care physicians and specialists at PHC clinics, and improved coordination with the hospital sector and the health insurance system.

Study on the Medical Standards, Quality and Appropriateness of Health Services in Hospitals and Primary Health Care Providers

Due to the varied backgrounds of the medical personnel, the lack of medical standards and procedures, and the limited capacity in the system to monitor the quality of service, there is evidence of problems in the quality of medical care in the WBG. This study will investigate in detail the medical practices in hospitals and primary care services to identify the major problems in terms of the quality appropriateness of: diagnosis, treatment and medical procedures, referrals and laboratory procedures. The study will include the analysis of available data on case-specific utilization patterns on hospitals and primary care clinics and will be supplemented by data collected at the facilities through observational studies (e.g., time-and-motion study); interviews of medical personnel regarding the common medical practice, qualifications, knowledge of medical procedures; and review of medical records.

Information collected from these data will be synthesized to identify major problem areas requiring special attention, e.g., performance of unnecessary surgery, overprescription of particular drugs, inappropriate referrals, etc. For example, the very short length of stay in government hospitals suggests the likelihood of unnecessary admissions in hospitals. This study will furnish qualitative data on medical practices and quality of services at government, private and NGO hospitals and clinics. These data could be used to develop future medical education and continuing education program for medical personnel; promote the establishment of quality improvement programs through the key professional associations (e.g., medical, hospital and pharmaceutical associations); set standards for licensing requirements; and establish a basic information and monitoring system for quality regulation by the MOH. In addition, these data will be compared with population-based epidemiological data to ensure that the health services are meeting the priority health needs of the population.

INFRASTRUCTURE INVESTMENT PLAN: TERMS OF REFERENCE

Health system in the West Bank and Gaza is a complex amalgam of providers including MOH, UNRWA, NGOs and an emerging private sector. Investment in health infrastructure calls for assessment of number of facilities available and their utilization pattern across all sub-sectors, consideration of the demographic and epidemiological characteristics of the population, and also of existing resources available. Design of facilities in terms of allocation of space, relative proximity of services and appropriateness for medical equipment also needs to be considered.

Rationalization of investment will require (i) development of institutional capacity of planning units in public sector (ii) development of a facility and equipment masterplan based on revised norms and standards.

SUGGESTED SCOPE OF WORK

Contribution from Palestinian Authority

- Formation of Core Group consisting of representatives from Planning and Policy Making Council and other sub-sectors such as UNRWA, NGOs and private providers who are familiar with facility planning and needs assessments. Its function would be to quantify the need for health services, and identify appropriate facility and equipment norms and standards. It would also follow up on activities of the Task Group.

- Formation of Task Group, whose members will be drawn from health ministry from amongst those who are working in planning [e.g. department of planning], facility management [e.g. hospital director], construction and maintenance. They will undergo training by technical specialists and be responsible for, collecting and analyzing the relevant data, development of health services map, assisting in the formulation and application of norms and standards, and managing the implementation of outcomes.

- Organization of a study tour to observe the effect of applying criteria and standards developed to facilities and equipment.

- Organizing and making arrangements for training workshops

- Provision of available data and information and transportation for data collection teams.

- Organization of meeting at completion, for presentation of findings to National Health Committee and relevant ministries [e.g. Health, Planning, etc.], with inclusion from various sub-sectors such as UNRWA.

Contribution from Technical Specialist Team

- Work with the Core Group to develop criteria and indicators to be used to quantify the need for health services, and appropriate facility and equipment norms and standards.

- Train Task Group in collection of relevant data on which to quantify demand and measure the degree of compliance to norms and standards.

- Initiate preparations for the training workshops and provide training

- Initiate planning for the study tour

- Further expand the health services map, developed by the Department of Planning at MOH, to incorporates data on existing equipment and facilities and serve as a tool to identify priority areas for future investment.

- Present findings, conclusions and recommendations at meeting of National Health Planning Committee, other relevant ministries and UNRWA.

- Institutionalize the preparation of sound investment strategies which maximize through staff training, codifying norms and standards, preparing conceptual designs and developing databases for synthesizing information collected.

DATA FOR HUMAN RESOURCES DEVELOPMENT

The following are data which should be collected across the various providers and payers and made available at various levels to people involved in policy, organization, management and delivery of services. It can be especially useful in the development of a human resources masterplan and its implementation in the West Bank and Gaza.

Environment of the Health Care System

Actors involved.

- interested groups (government ministries and departments, UNRWA, NGOs, and private sector, political groups, professional syndicates, associations, training institutions, students/teachers associations, unions, research agencies, consumers representatives)
- their views and objectives and their relative influence

These can be collected through the analysis of policy statements, recommendations of official reports and other relevant reports (research, UNRWA, NGOs, donor agencies, professional associations, etc.) and through surveys.

Legal framework.

- all laws and regulations related to health and population human resources
- administrative/institutional framework of public services
- economic trends
- resources available for training, employing health personnel

Stock of providers.

- distribution by category of establishments; hospitals, health centers, polyclinics, individual clinics
- distribution by type of activities (clinical - public and private, administrative, teaching); time devoted to each type of activity (information needed to calculate full-time equivalence)
- distribution by level of training
- distribution by level of activity: in training, at work, not employed
- geographical distribution; by governorate; rural/urban
- distribution by age, gender, other available socio-demographic variables
- ratios: population/provider, provider/provider (e.g.: nurse/doctor, specialist/generalist), government/private, NGOs, UNRWA
- human resource dynamics: entries, migration, attrition; human resource trends
- training (number and type of schools, intake capacity, real intake, attrition, number of graduates, duration of programs, contents, quality, training abroad, teaching staff, curricula, teaching methods, admission procedures) and development (continuing education, in-service training)
- recruitment, posting, transfer, promotion, career plans (mobility of personnel);

- definition of duties and responsibilities (job description, workload, under/over-utilization)
- working conditions (including pay)
- supervision and evaluation
- system of incentives (financial and others) which must be related to financing of the sector

Services and Facilities (actual and projected)

- number of establishments by category; hospitals, health centers, polyclinics, individual clinics
- number of establishments by level of service delivery (primary, secondary, tertiary)
- geographical distribution of establishments; by region; rural/urban
- number of establishments by source of funding (government - MOH, UNRWA, other ministries; donors; private; NGOs)
- establishments by size (number of clinical and non-clinical posts)
- costs by budget chapter
- function, structure of establishments; functional links

Appendix 8: ORGANIZATIONAL STRUCTURE OF MINISTRY OF HEALTH

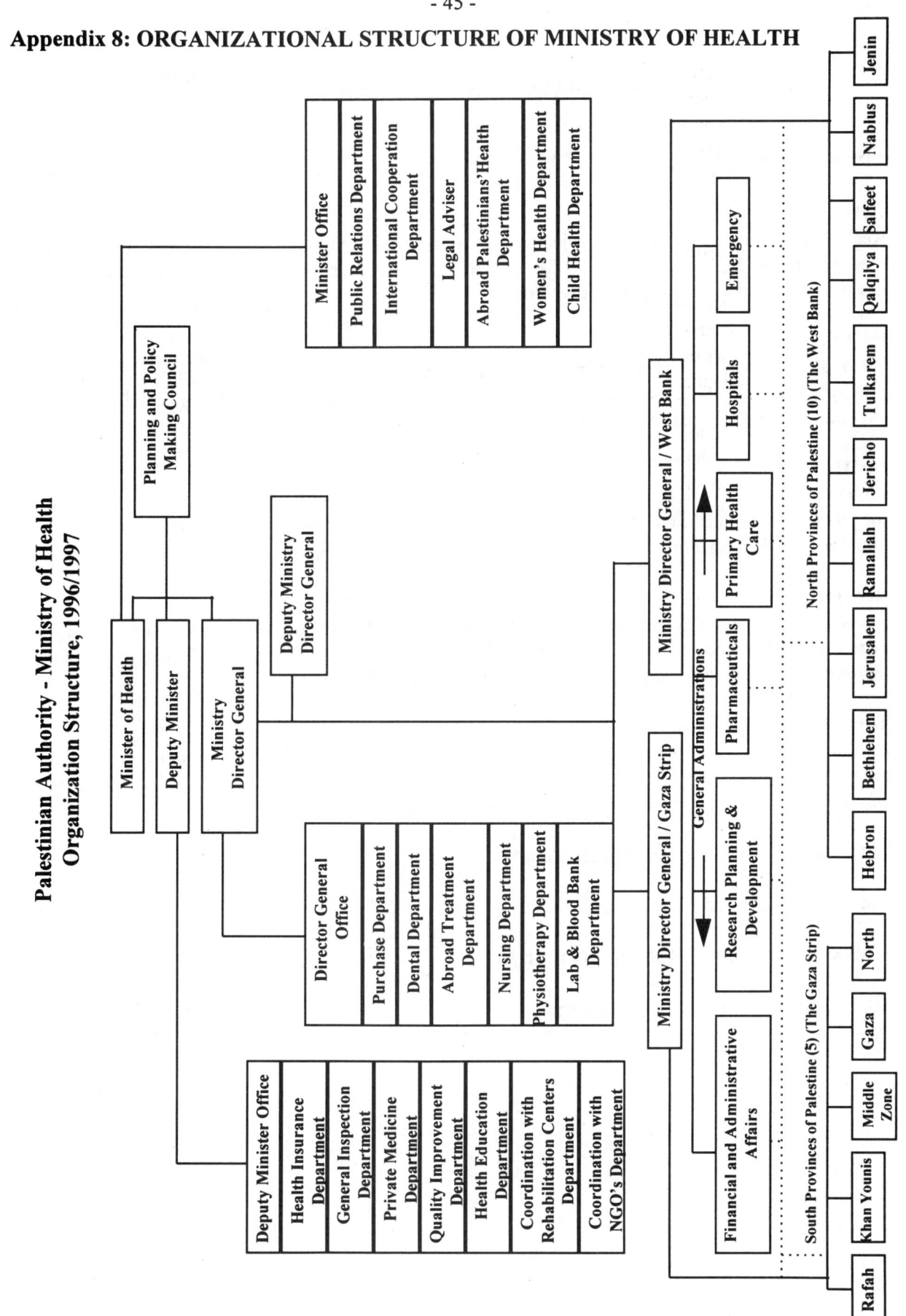

Palestinian Authority - Ministry of Health
Organization Structure, 1996/1997

Appendix 9: MACROECONOMIC PROJECTIONS

METHOD OF CALCULATION

GDP:

Real GDP at constant prices was projected assuming annual growth rates at low GDP growth for scenario 1 and higher GDP growth for scenario 2. GDP at current prices was calculated by multiplying GDP at constant prices with deflator.

PA Budget:

PA budget in terms of revenue, current PA expenditure, public investment and foreign financed program was given for 1997 and worked out to be 23% of the GDP. We assumed that PA expenditure would remain at the same proportion of GDP for the next five years.

MOH Budget:

MOH revenue and current expenditure as percentage of PA revenue and expenditure was given for 1997. We assumed that MOH budget would remain constant during the next five year period with the only incremental increase being that of recurrent cost of investments.

Recurrent Costs:

Recurrent cost estimates were provided for the entire period based on MOH Investment Plan for Scenario 1 and Recommended Investment Plan for Scenario 2. They are shown as annual incremental expenditure and also expressed as percentage of MOH expenditure.

Total MOH Expenditures:

In order to have a full picture of the MOH expenditures, we added up the annual incremental recurrent expenditure to the MOH budget. The total MOH expenditure was then expressed as percentage of GDP and percentage of total PA expenditure.

SCENARIOS A: HIGHER RECURRENT COSTS

See Scenarios A1 and A2 in Pages 2 and 3.

SCENARIOS B: LOWER RECURRENT COSTS

See Scenarios B1 and B2 in Pages 4 and 5.

Table A2.2: Total Investment 1997-9002 in Accordance with
Ministry of Health Priorities, June 1997

(US$ million) West Bank and Gaza including European Union	1997	1998	1999	1998	2001	2002	Cumulative
Hospital Investment	35.87	35.87	35.87	35.87	35.87	35.87	**215.2**
Recurrent Cost 20 Percent	0	7.17	14.35	21.52	28.69	35.87	107.60
Recurrent Cost 25 Percent	0	8.97	17.93	26.90	35.87	44.83	134.50
Recurrent Cost 30 Percent	0	10.76	21.52	32.28	43.04	53.80	161.40
PHC Investment	11.1	8.5	8.5	6.9	4.2	4	**43.1**
Recurrent Cost 30 Percent	0	3.3	5.9	8.4	10.5	11.8	39.9
Recurrent Cost 40 Percent	0	4.44	7.84	11.24	14	15.68	53.2
Other Investment							
I. Ambulance Services	0.83	0.83	0.83	0.83	0.83	0.83	5.00
II. Buildings							
Public Health Laboratory	0.47	0.47	0.47	0.47	0.47	0.47	2.80
Laundry Building	0.04	0.04	0.04	0.04	0.04	0.04	0.25
Nursing School	0.25	0.25	0.25	0.25	0.25	0.25	1.50
Central Stores	0.42	0.42	0.42	0.42	0.42	0.42	2.50
Maintenance Workshop	0.04	0.04	0.04	0.04	0.04	0.04	0.25
Sub Total Buildings	1.22	1.22	1.22	1.22	1.22	1.22	7.30
Total Other Investments							12.30
Recurrent Cost of Other							
Ambulance 15 Percent	0	0.12	0.31	0.49	0.67	0.85	2.45
Miscellaneous Buildings 5 Percent	0	0.06	0.12	0.18	0.24	0.30	0.91
Total Investment Cost	49.02	46.42	46.42	44.82	42.12	41.92	270.60
Total Recurrent Expenditure	0.00	10.69	20.66	30.62	40.11	48.79	150.86

Note: Hospital and PHC investment costs include cost of infrastructure, rehabilitation and equipment as listed by MOH priorities, June 1997.

Recurrent cost for hospital sector [in terms of salaries, supplies, etc.] also includes operating cost of EU hospital presently under construction. Capital cost of EU Hospital has not been included as it is assumed to be supported by EU and UNRWA.

Total recurrent cost calculated using hospital cost @ 20% of investment, PHC @ 30% and recurrent cost of other investments as their given rates. Rates for calculation of recurrent cost vary from 20 - 33% for hospitals and are higher for smaller facilities.

Source: M. Hopkinson and K. Kostermans, <u>Building for Health Care</u>, World Bank 1996.

Scenario #A1: Low Case

Real GDP growth rate: negative or equal to zero
Pa revenue: decrease/GDP   Pa expenditure: same proportion/GDP

MOH revenue: same proportion/PA revenue   MOH expenditure: same proportion/PA expenditure

	1997	1998	1999	2000	2001	2002
Assumptions						
Real GDP (growth rate)	5.4%	-1.0%	-1.0%	-0.5%	0%	0%
Real GDP (constant prices)	1,154	1,142	1,131	1,125	1,125	1,125
GDP (current prices)	3,546	3,795	4,061	4,405	4,801	5,233
Deflator	3.07	3.32	3.59	3.91	4.27	4.65
iInlation	8%	8%	8%	9%	9%	9%
PA Budget						
Revenue	814	759	731	749	768	785
Current Ependiture	866	911	975	1057	1152	1256
Current Deficit	-52	-152	-244	-308	-384	-471
Public Investment	255	228	244	264	288	314
Foreign Financed Program	0	0	0	0	0	0
Overall Deficit (percentage of GDP)	-307	-379	-487	-573	-672	-785
Revenue	23	20	18	17	16	15
Current Expenditure	24	24	24	24	24	24
Current Deficit	-1	-4	-6	-7	-8	-9
Public Investment	7	6	6	6	6	6
Foreign Financed Program	0	0	0	0	0	0
Overall Deficit	-9	-10	-12	-13	-14	-15
MOH Budget						
Revenue	30.91	30.36	29.24	29.95	30.73	31.40
Current Expenditure	96.94	100.19	107.22	116.28	126.75	138.16
Current Deficit (percentage of PA budget)	-66.03	-69.83	-77.98	-86.33	-96.02	-106.76
Revenue	4	4	4	4	4	4
Current Expenditure	11	11	11	11	11	11

Public Investment Plan and Recurrent Cost Implications for the Health Sector, 1997 - 2002						
Public Investment Plan	0	0	0	0	0	0
Recurrent cost estimates						
Projection I (high)	0.00	10.69	20.66	30.62	40.11	48.79
Total	0.00	10.69	20.66	30.62	40.11	48.79
Total 1 (as % of MOH current expenditure)	0%	11%	19%	26%	32%	35%

Result In the low case scenario, these additional investments and recurrent costs will represent up to 35 percent of the MOH current expenditure at the end of the period.

Total MOH expenditure						
Total	96.94	110.88	127.88	146.90	166.86	186.95
as percentage of GDP						
Total I	2.7%	2.9%	3.1%	3.3%	3.5%	3.6%
as percentage of PA total expenditure						
Total I	8.6%	9.7%	10.5%	11.1%	11.6%	11.9%

Result in the low case scenario, MOH total expenditure represent about 3.6% of GDP and up to 12% of PA total expenditure.

Scenario #A2: Medium Case
Real GDP growth rate: lower than case #1
Pa revenue: lower than case #1   Pa expenditure: same proportion/GDP
MOH revenue: same proportion/PA revenue   MOH expenditure: same proportion/PA expenditure

	1997	1998	1999	2000	2001	2002
Assumptions						
Real GDP (growth rate)	5.4%	2.0%	2.5%	3.3%	3.5%	3.5%
Real GDP (constant prices)	1,154	1,177	1,206	1,246	1,289	1,334
GDP (current prices)	3,546	3,910	4,332	4,876	5,500	6,205
Deflator	3.07	3.32	3.59	3.91	4.27	4.65
Inflation	8%	8%	8%	9%	9%	9%
PA Budget						
Revenue	814	841	910	1024	1155	1272
Current Expenditure	866	938	1040	1170	1320	1489
Current Deficit	-52	-98	-130	-146	-165	-217
Public Investment	255	235	260	293	330	372
Foreign Financed Program	0	0	0	0	0	0
Overall Deficit (percentage of GDP)	-307	-332	-390	-439	-495	-590
Revenue	23	22	21	21	21	21
Current Expenditure	24	24	24	24	24	24
Current Deficit	-1	-3	-3	-3	-3	-4
Public Investment	7	6	6	6	6	6
Foreign Financed Program	0	0	0	0	0	0
Overall Deficit	-9	-9	-9	-9	-9	-10
MOH Budget						
Revenue	30.91	33.63	36.39	40.96	46.20	50.88
Current Expenditure	96.94	103.22	114.37	128.72	145.21	163.82
Current deficit (percentage of PA Budget)	-66.03	-69.60	-77.98	-87.76	-99.01	-112.94
Revenue	4	4	4	4	4	4
Current Expenditure	11	11	11	11	11	11

Public Investment Plan and Recurrent Cost Implications for the Health Sector, 1997 - 2002						
Public Investment Plan	0	0	0	0	0	0
Recurrent Cost Estimates						
	0.00	10.69	20.66	30.62	40.11	48.79
Total	0.00	10.69	20.66	30.62	40.11	48.79
Total 1 (% of MOH current expenditure)	0	10	18	24	28	30

Result In the low case scenario, these additional investments and recurrent costs will represent up to 30 percent of the MOH current expenditure at the end of the period.

Total MOH Expenditure						
	96.94	113.91	135.03	159.34	185.32	212.61
As Percentage of GDP						
	2.7	2.9	3.1	3.3	3.4	3.4
As Percentage of PA total Expenditure						
	8.6	9.7	10.4	10.9	11.2	11.4

Result in the medium case scenario, MOH total expenditure represent about 3.4% of GDP and up to 11.4% of PA total expenditure.

Scenario #B1: Low Case						
Real GDP growth rate: negative or equal to zero						
Pa revenue: decrease/GDP Pa expenditure: same proportion/GDP						
MOH revenue: same proportion/PA revenue MOH expenditure: same proportion/PA expenditure						
	1997	**1998**	**1999**	**2000**	**2001**	**2002**
Assumptions						
Real GDP (growth rate)	5.4%	-1.0%	-1.0%	-0.5%	0%	0%
Real GDP (constant prices)	1,154	1,142	1,131	1,125	1,125	1,125
GDP (current prices)	3,546	3,795	4,061	4,405	4,801	5,233
Deflator	3.07	3.32	3.59	3.91	4.27	4.65
Inflation	8%	8%	8%	9%	9%	9%
PA Budget						
Revenue	814	759	731	749	768	785
Current Expenditure	866	911	975	1057	1152	1256
Current Deficit	-52	-152	-244	-308	-384	-471
Public Investment	255	228	244	264	288	314
Foreign Financed Program	0	0	0	0	0	0
Overall Deficit (percentage of GDP)	-307	-379	-487	-573	-672	-785
Revenue	*23*	20	18	17	16	15
Current Expenditure	*24*	24	24	24	24	24
Current Deficit	*-1*	-4	-6	-7	-8	-9
Public Investment	*7*	6	6	6	6	6
Foreign Financed Program	*0*	0	0	0	0	0
Overall Deficit	*-9*	-10	-12	-13	-14	-15
MOH Budget						
Revenue	30.91	30.36	29.24	29.95	30.73	31.40
Current Expenditure	96.94	100.19	107.22	116.28	126.75	138.16
Current Deficit (percentage of PA budget)	-66.03	-69.83	-77.98	-86.33	-96.02	-106.76
Revenue	4	4	4	4	4	4
Current expenditure	11	11	11	11	11	11

Public Investment Plan and Recurrent Cost Implications for the Health Sector, 1997 - 2002						
Public Investment Plan	0	0	0	0	0	0
Recurrent Cost Estimates						
Projection I (high)	0.00	8.64	16.55	24.47	31.90	38.53
Total	0.00	8.64	16.55	24.47	31.90	38.53
Total 1 (% of MOH current expenditure)	**0**	**9**	**15**	**21**	**25**	**28**
Result In the low case scenario, these additional investments and recurrent costs will represent up to 28 percent of the MOH current expenditure at the end of the period.						
Total MOH Expenditure	96.94	108.83	123.77	140.75	158.65	176.69
As Percentage of GDP	2.7	2.9	3.0	3.2	3.3	3.4
As Percentage of PA Total Expenditure	8.6	9.6	10.2	10.7	11.0	11.3
Result in the low case scenario, MOH total expenditure represent about 3.4% of GDP and up to 11.3% of PA total expenditure.						

Scenario #B2: Medium Case						
Real GDP growth rate: lower than case #1						
Pa revenue: lower than case #1		Pa expenditure: same proportion/GDP				
MOH revenue: same proportion/PA revenue		MOH expenditure: same proportion/PA expenditure				
	1997	**1998**	**1999**	**2000**	**2001**	**2002**
Assumptions						
Real GDP (growth rate)	5.4%	2.0%	2.5%	3.3%	3.5%	3.5%
Real GDP (constant prices)	1,154	1,177	1,206	1,246	1,289	1,334
GDP (current prices)	3,546	3,910	4,332	4,876	5,500	6,205
Deflator	3.07	3.32	3.59	3.91	4.27	4.65
Inflation	8%	8%	8%	9%	9%	9%
PA Budget						
Revenue	814	841	910	1024	1155	1272
Current Expenditure	866	938	1040	1170	1320	1489
Current Deficit	-52	-98	-130	-146	-165	-217
Public Investment	255	235	260	293	330	372
Foreign Financed Program	0	0	0	0	0	0
Overall Deficit (percentage of GDP)	-307	-332	-390	-439	-495	-590
Revenue	*23*	22	21	21	21	21
Current Expenditure	*24*	24	24	24	24	24
Current Deficit	*-1*	-3	-3	-3	-3	-4
Public Investment	7	6	6	6	6	6
Foreign Financed Program	*0*	0	0	0	0	0
Overall Deficit	*-9*	-9	-9	-9	-9	-10
MOH Budget						
Revenue	30.91	33.63	36.39	40.96	46.20	50.88
Current Expenditure	96.94	103.22	114.37	128.72	145.21	163.82
Current deficit (percentage of PA budget)	-66.03	-69.60	-77.98	-87.76	-99.01	-112.94
Revenue	4	4	4	4	4	4
Current Expenditure	11	11	11	11	11	11

Public Investment Plan and Recurrent Cost Implications for the Health Sector, 1997 - 2002						
Public Investment Plan	0	0	0	0	0	0
Recurrent Cost Estimates						
	0.00	8.64	16.55	24.47	31.90	38.53
Total	0.00	8.64	16.55	24.47	31.90	38.53
Total 1 (% of MOH Current Expenditure)	**0**	**8**	**14**	**19**	**22**	**24**
Result In the low case scenario, these additional investments and recurrent costs will represent up to 61 percent of the MOH current expenditure at the end of the period.						
Total MOH Expenditure	96.94	111.86	130.92	153.19	177.11	202.35
As Percentage of GDP	2.7	2.9	3.0	3.1	3.2	3.3
As Percentage of PA Total Expenditure	8.6	9.5	10.1	10.5	10.7	10.9
Result in the medium case scenario, MOH total expenditure represent about 3.3% of GDP and up to 10.9% of PA total expenditure.						

Appendix 10: WORKING PAPER ON FINANCING AND ORGANIZATION OF HEALTH SERVICES

INTRODUCTION

This paper has been prepared as part of the Health Sector Study for the West Bank and Gaza (WBG) conducted jointly by the Ministry of Health (MOH), World Health Organization (WHO) and the World Bank in May 1997. The paper focuses on issues related to health financing, and aims to :

- update and synthesize the latest available information on health financing, including a flow of funds analysis and, where possible, unit cost analysis;

- examine the salient trends in health financing and analyze their implications on the short and medium-term development of the health system in terms of (a) affordability (sustainability), (b) quality and efficiency, and (c) equity;

- estimate the projected revenue and expenditure patterns for the MOH under different policy scenarios; and

- identify areas that require urgent action to address the imminent financial crisis in the health sector, and suggest some longer-term health financing policies that would support the development of an efficient and equitable health system.

A team from the World Bank visited the WBG from May 6 - May 22, 1997. The analyses presented herein are based on the available studies and reports as well as information collected by the team during the visits to various offices of the MOH in WBG; hospitals and health centers in the government, non-governmental and private sectors; UN and other donor agencies; non-governmental organization (NGO) representatives and a number of individuals in the private sector involved in the health sector in the WBG; and the Palestinian Central Statistical Bureau. The list of persons met by the mission are provided in Annex 1; the main references are listed in Annex 2.

With regard to data analysis in this report, two points of clarification are worth mentioning. First, an estimation of health financing in per capita terms or as a percentage of GDP is subject to significant variation because of the considerable uncertainties in the key demographic and macroeconomic figures for the WBG. Unless otherwise indicated, the population and macroeconomic figures shown in Table A 10.1 are used throughout this paper. Some discrepancies in health financing figures between the estimates provided in this paper and other previously published papers might occur due to these differences in the choice of population and macroeconomic figures.

Secondly, in this paper East Jerusalem is treated as a separate entity from WBG. Readers are cautioned that some of the published reports include East Jerusalem in the aggregate analyses of WBG. This could result in some discrepancies between the numbers cited in this report and those of previously published reports.

Table A 10.1: Macroeconomic and Demographic Indicators for West Bank and Gaza

	1993	1994	1995	1996
GDP, US$ million	2,557	3,077	3,222	3,233
GNP, US$ million	3,109	3,463	3,469	3,438
Population, total	1,901	2,015	2,151	2,280
West Bank	1,113	1,172	1,246	1,317
Gaza Strip	788	843	905	963

Sources: GDP and GNP figures are from International Monetary Fund (IMF), "Recent Economic Developments, Prospects, and Progress in Institution Building in the West Bank and Gaza Strip", Middle Eastern Department, 1997. The population figures are World Bank estimates (1997), which excludes the East Jerusalem population.

The report is divided into five sections: Section II provides an overview of the trends in health financing in the WBG, including a discussion on the government policies in the health sector; Section III provides a more detailed analysis of the various components of the health financing system based on the latest available data; Section IV evaluates the performance of the existing health financing system in terms of (a) affordability and sustainability, (b) efficiency and quality of care, and (c) equity and access to care; and Section V will conclude with suggestions for a number options for actions and policies to improve the performance of the health financing system in the short, medium-term and long-term.

HEALTH FINANCING IN WEST BANK AND GAZA: RECENT TRENDS

General Trends: 1994-1997

Just three years have passed since the Palestinian Authority (PA) assumed the responsibility of managing and financing the health service sector from the Israeli Civil Administration. The health system that has evolved in that short period reflects both the features inherited from the Civil Administration as well as the aspects introduced by the newly established MOH.

Prior to the handover, the notable features of the health financing system included: (a) a heavy reliance on external assistance and NGO contributions for a significant part of health financing (over 40 percent in 1991, including UNRWA), (b) relatively limited contributions from the government (i.e., Civil Administration), derived primarily from health insurance premium, that covered less than a fifth of total health expenditure and only about a fifth of the Palestinian population, and (c) direct household expenditures that accounted for about 40 percent of the total health expenditures.

Since the handover, the following critical changes have occurred in the overall health financing system:

- While the basic structure of the Government Health Insurance (GHI) system has been retained, premium levels were reduced significantly to encourage the expansion of coverage. This had reduced the ratio of premium revenues to expenditure and the difference has been increasingly made up through budgetary allocations from the government's general tax revenues. In net effect, the financing of government health system has shifted from one based on social insurance to a system based primarily on general tax revenues, with supplementary revenues from health insurance premium payments.

- Donor contributions continue to be an important source of revenues for the health sector, but the main recipient of aid has shifted from the NGO sector to MOH. The substance of donor assistance has also changed from budgetary support for the delivery of health services to a greater emphasis on capital investments, training and other developmental activities aimed at expanding the capacity of the government health delivery system. For the NGO sector, this loss of revenues has not been compensated by an inflow of funds from the other sectors. For example, since the GHI only covers tertiary services, it does not reimburse many services provided by the NGOs and thus many NGO providers have not benefited from the expansion in insurance coverage.

- UNRWA continues to provide free basic health services for the refugee population. Although donor contributions to UNRWA swelled in the early 1990s, the budget is no longer keeping up with the rapid refugee population growth rate.

- Private investors are entering the market primarily at the high technology end of health services (diagnostic centers polyclinics and specialty hospitals). Private practitioners, however, remain largely unorganized as a group, although the expansion in the for-profit clinics and hospitals may provide a focal point for future organization of medical practitioners.

- While actual enrollment figures are not available, private health insurance coverage appears to be very limited. A number of local insurance companies that began offering health insurance plans in the last two years appear to be experiencing problems typical of nascent insurance markets (moral hazard and selection bias). Predictably, these companies are beginning to introduce measures to select out the high risk population in order to maintain financial solvency.

Table A 10.2 summarizes the national health expenditure patterns by sources of revenue for the years 1991 and 1995-97. These figures should be treated only as indicative figures, particularly because of the uncertainties in the size of the NGO sector. Data on contributions from private corporations for their employee health care are also missing. The slight increase in the health expenditure to GDP ratio from 1995 to 1996 can be attributed to a slowdown in the overall economic growth rate rather than to a significant increase in health expenditure. Total health expenditures for 1995-97 include public and private capital investments.

Using the GDP and population figures shown in Table A 10.1, the total health expenditure is estimated to be around 9 percent of GDP. By international standards this is a relatively high level of health expenditure for countries at a comparable income level: middle income countries typically spend between 4 to 6 percent of GDP on health care. It should be emphasized that part of this high level of spending has been supported by the substantial donor assistance: on average donor contributions accounted for about 12 percent of the total health spending between 1995-97.

Table A 10.2: National Health Expenditures in West Bank and Gaza, 1991-97
(US$, millions, unless otherwise indicated)

	1991	1995	1996	1997 *(projected)*
Total GDP	~ 2,600	3,222	3,233	Not Available
Health Expenditure as Percent of GDP	~ 9	8.690	8.6	Not Available
Per Capita Health Expenditure (US$)	Not Available/[1]	$125	~ $122	~ $111
Total Health Expenditure /[2]	224	276	~ 278	~ 263
Government Health Insurance	42	24	22	27 /[3]
General Revenues	-	45	67	61
UNRWA	13	29	23	30
Donors	77 /[4]	33	44	31
NGOs	-	37	~ 20 ? /[5]	~ 10 ? /[5]
Private /[6]	91	108	102	105

Notes: 1. The per capita figure is not shown for this year because of the very large uncertainties in the population size.
2. Includes capital expenditures, except for 1991.
3. Based on revenues in the first half of the 1997 financial year.
4. This figure combines the contributions from international donors and NGOs.
5. NGO contributions for 1996 and 1997 are not available. The figures shown are rough estimations based on the assumption that NGO contributions have been shrinking steadily during these years.
6. Private expenditure includes household expenditure on health care, MOH copayments and private capital investments, but excludes household payments for government insurance premium.
Sources: 1991 figures are from The World Bank, "Developing the Occupied Territories," Vol. 6, 1993; 1995 figures are based on Barghouti and Lennock; and 1996,1997 figures are World Bank staff estimates based on data collected during the study. See Appendix 11 for details.

Table A 10.3: National Health Expenditures in West Bank and Gaza, 1991-97
(percent distribution by sources of revenues)

Source	1991	1995	1996	1997
Government Health Insurance	19	9	8	10
General Revenues	0	17	24	23
UNRWA	6	11	8	11
Donor Contributions	34	9	16	12
NGOs	0	14	7	4
Private	41	40	37	40
Total	100	100	100	100

Source: Table A 10.2, above.

IMPACT OF BORDER CLOSURES AND ECONOMIC DIFFICULTIES, 1996-97

The frequent border closures and political uncertainties that marked the year 1996 resulted in severe disruptions to the economy and a sharp rise in unemployment rates. These events could not have come at a more inopportune moment in the development of the Palestinian health system. Health sector investment plans prepared in the early days of the PA were designed to achieve a rapid expansion of the health system under the assumption of a relatively stable economic growth (see National Health Plan 1994). Many of the investments in the new health facilities are about to come on stream at a time when resources to operate these new facilities are declining. Moreover, these closures impede the movement of goods and services as well as health staff and patients to and from the health facilities, and create shortages and delays in ongoing constructions projects. The deteriorating economic conditions also present a serious set back to PA's plans to expand social insurance coverage, since the success of such policies requires steady economic growth and an expanding formal employment sector. Figure A 10.1 illustrates the impact of closures on the flow of revenues from health insurance premium, as households appear to withhold payments during times of economic hardship.

Figure A 10.1: Impact of Border Closures on the Government Health Insurance

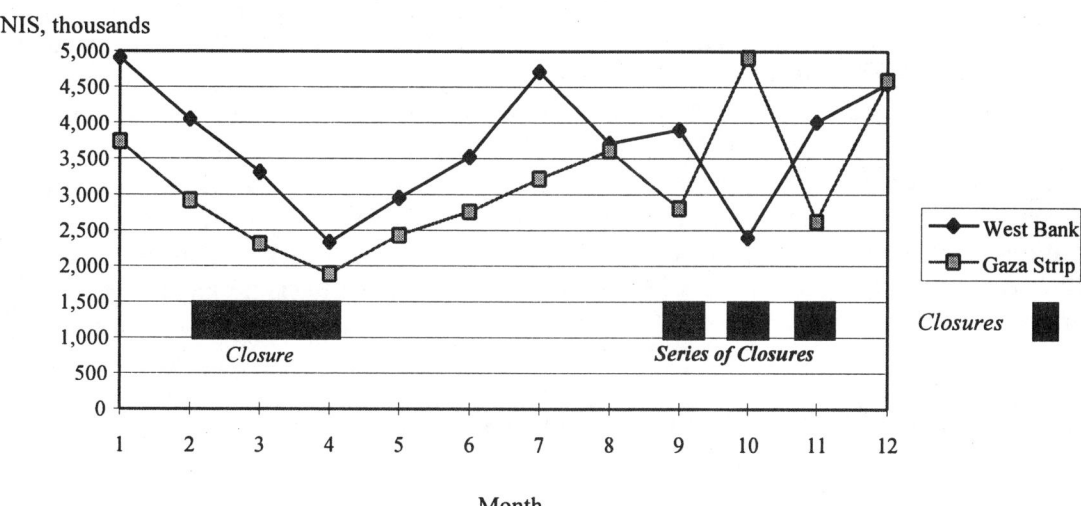

Government Health Insurance - Monthly Premium Revenues, 1996

Source: Health Insurance Department, Ministry of Health, Gaza City, 1997.

GOVERNMENT POLICIES ON HEALTH FINANCING, 1994-96

Expansion of the Government Health System

At the time of its inception in 1994, the Health Council, and subsequently the MOH, has accorded the highest priority to the expansion of the health insurance coverage and access to health care services to the Palestinian population. This is reflected in the 1994 National Health Plan which laid out an investment strategy to compensate for years of underinvestment in the health services during the years of occupation. In the last two years, the MOH has been relatively successful in: (a) achieving a significant expansion in health insurance coverage and in maintaining the system of revenue collection inherited from the Israeli Civil Administration; (b) organizing a centralized budgeting, procurement and distribution system to finance and manage a growing network of public providers; and (c) managing a system of subcontracting from health care providers mainly to through overseas providers, and increasingly to providers within the WBG. These achievements are not trivial given the very short time in which they have been implemented.

PA's commitment to the expansion of the health delivery system is evident from the sizable allocation of government revenues to the MOH (Table A 10.4). Health insurance is included as part of the government budget since all revenues from insurance premiums are transferred directly to the Ministry of Finance (MOF), and reallocated to MOH as part of the budget appropriations process. Despite recent economic difficulties, total government revenues have shown a strong growth over the period of 1995-97 due to the significant improvements in tax administration during this period. PA supported a nearly 30 percent increase in health budget for 1996, of which most of the increase came from the general revenues.

The pro-expansion policies of the past two years are generating a momentum towards cost-escalation. They include: (a) the expansion of health insurance coverage which will raise the per capita utilization of health services as additional households gain financial access to services through insurance (moral hazard); (b) a growing supply of health care services, particularly through the planned expansion of acute care bed capacities (by as much as 50 percent over existing capacity - see Annex 9) which will raise utilization rates as well as incur additional fixed operating and capital costs; (c) the introduction of major technology upgrades within the existing public hospitals as well as the encouragement of private investments in facilities equipped with advanced medical technology; (e) a rapid rise in the consumption of drugs (a jump from 22 percent of total expenditure in 1995 to about 32 percent in 1997 in the government sector alone) promoted by a policy of providing ready access to a plethora of drugs (see the Pharmaceutical Sector Report); and (e) a generous policy of subsidizing overseas treatment for cases which cannot be treated within the WBG. Moreover, the underlying epidemiological changes and rapid population growth rates will create a strong demand for health services in the coming decades. The government continues to support a public investment program which will substantially expand the MOH health delivery capacity over the next five years.

Table A 10.4: Total Government Revenues and Health Budget, 1995-97
(US$ million)

Budget Category	1995	1996	1997 (projection)
Government Revenues	425	670	814
MOH Budget	69	89	88
- From General Revenues	45	67	61
- From Health Insurance Premium	24	22	27
MOH Budget (including insurance premium) as Percent of Total Government Revenues	16	13	11

Sources: Government revenues are IMF estimates (see IMF, 1997); the MOH budget data were provided by MOH, Gaza and Nablus, 1997.

Cost containment and rationalization of resource use

The worsening economic situation will impose a global constraint on the growth in government financing of health services in the coming years. The effects are likely to be felt more immediately through the retrenchment in revenues from the health insurance premiums, reflecting the sensitivities of household income to border closures and rising unemployment rates. The shortfall from health insurance revenues could be partially compensated by an increase in budget allocation from general revenues, but according to at least one MOH projection the total MOH budget (including health insurance) for 1997 might fall below the 1996 level[58]. These fiscal problems are compounded this year by delays in the budget approval process by the Legislative Council. As of May 1997 all ministries were continuing to operate at the 1996 budget levels, with the notable exception of the MOH which has been permitted selective increases over its 1996 budget to accommodate the previously planned expansion in government health services.

In response to these fiscal uncertainties, the MOH has begun to introduce some measures that focus on efficiency gains and cost containment. Since 1996 the Ministry has started restricting the number of referrals to the Israeli hospitals -- which are several times more costly than referrals to providers in Jordan or Egypt. To control the rising expenditure on drugs, the Ministry is currently developing an essential drugs policy which will be introduced shortly. Preparatory work is also underway -- with technical assistance from a variety of donor agencies -- to improve the efficiency and quality of medical services, including a cost analysis of hospital

---

[58] The recent restriction to Palestinian tax revenues collected by the Israeli authorities could affect budget allocations

services, the establishment of standards and protocols for effective and efficient clinical procedures, and the introduction of Quality Improvement Program to strengthen the management of health services. Cost containment policies are also producing some adverse effects. For example, salary increases have been held down in recent years to the extent that they are beginning to have a negative impact on staff morale and quality of care. On the whole, measures to rationalize the use of resources appear to be somewhat fragmented and could benefit from a more coherent and strategic policy framework.

Policies toward private providers

The MOH has been encouraging private investments in the health delivery system as a means of expanding the total health service capacity within the WBG, promoting competition, and reducing the number of overseas treatments. Because priority is given to reducing the number of overseas treatment, MOH generally confines the purchase of services to tertiary care and advanced diagnostics services which are not available at the government hospitals.

With regard to secondary and primary care services, the MOH has pursued a policy of expanding services to the population through its own public delivery rather than by extending the purchasing arrangements with the existing private and NGO providers. One, possibly unintended, effect of this policy is to have encouraged private investments at the high technology end while restricting growth at the secondary level. The majority of the population have few alternatives to the GHI scheme, since the private health insurance is expensive and limited in scope. As a result, many NGO hospitals and clinics are currently facing financial difficulties because few patients have insurance coverage that reimburse them for the cost of hospitalization. This effect is also manifested in the relative under-utilization of the NGO hospitals (where bed occupancy rates are below the optimal capacity) while most government hospitals are operating at or above optimal capacity.

Private insurance market

To date, the private insurance market has received little attention from the MOH. There is a general perception among the MOH policy makers that because private health insurance covers mainly the well-to-do population, the government has a relatively little role to play in the sector. However, international experience shows that governments should have an interest in regulating the private insurance market for at least two reasons. First, a well-functioning private health insurance market can supplement the public financing of health services and increase the choice of providers and services for the patients. Secondly, by containing the negative effects of adverse selection among the competing private insurers, the government can play an important role in protecting social solidarity and ensuring a fair redistribution of resources for the poor. Private health insurance markets are highly susceptible to market failure problems, and in order to reduce these risks private insurers have very strong incentives to select out the high risk cases ("cherry-picking"). These adverse selection problems can lead to segmentation of the insurance market and to inequities in access to health care that are especially harmful for the poor. A well-designed regulatory regime can help to reduce the risk of failure for the insurers as well as mitigate the negative effects of adverse selection on equity.

The rules governing the use of government health services by privately insured patients are not clear. The MOH gives priority to patients covered under the GHI scheme, although patients without GHI coverage can be admitted into government hospitals if they pay the full fees. Patients injured in automobile accidents will have their hospitalization costs covered by their automobile insurance company, and the MOH collects the payments directly from the insurance companies. In principle, the MOH does not allow private insurance companies to purchase hospital services directly from government providers, but patients presumably have the option of being reimbursed retrospectively by their insurers for fees paid to the government health providers.

Universal coverage

As a long-term objective, the National Health Plan of 1994 proposed the development of a compulsory social insurance system as a means of achieving universal coverage. The Plan does not articulate this strategy beyond a very broad statement of objectives (see the report on Health Insurance Legislation). The policies and actions of the MOH since 1994 reveal a certain degree of ambivalence towards the implementation of this policy goal. First, the government health financing system has expanded largely in the direct provision of health services financed largely through general tax revenues (i.e., in the direction of an integrated health system typified by the National Health Service model of UK and the Scandinavian health systems) rather than through the expansion of the purchasing role of the GHI. Secondly, apart from the government employees and workers in Israel the enrollment in the GHI remains voluntary. For political reasons as well as in deference to the economic difficulties faced by households, the MOH has shown reluctance in imposing a compulsory system at this early stage in implementation. Policy makers should be aware that no country in the world has so far succeeded in achieving universal coverage by relying solely on voluntary participation. A voluntary insurance system tends to segment the market, and these tendencies toward fragmentation create major obstacles to universal coverage.

OVERVIEW OF THE HEALTH SYSTEM

An analysis of the health financing would be incomplete without an understanding of the overall organization of the health delivery system. The health system in the WBG can be broadly divided into three subsystems: the government sector, UNRWA, and NGO and private sector. The government sector is primarily defined by the system directly financed and operated by the MOH, although a separate smaller, health service program exists for the military and police, and some of the MOH services are purchased from overseas or from local private providers. An important characteristic of the public financing system that merits mentioning is that the revenues from various sources are collected into the single budget of the MOH. This distinguishes the Palestinian system from the other countries in the region (including Israel) which are dominated by a pluralistic health financing system. By retaining the structure of a single public financing agency, the Palestinian system avoids some of the inefficiencies and inequities associated with a pluralistic health financing system.

The distinction between "private" and "NGO" sectors is not well-defined: the NGO health providers, most of which were established during the occupation period through charitable donations, might be described as non-profit organizations although some appear to be developing into for-profit organizations. The Government purchases only a very limited selection of services from the NGO and private providers. UNRWA continues to operate independently to provide basic health services for the refugee population, but some of the UNRWA funds are also used to subcontract secondary services from the NGO hospitals for a limited number of refugee patients.

Figure in Appendix 1 presents an overview of the flow of funds from various sources to the health providers in different subsectors of the system.

Table A 10.5 describes the health systems in terms of the entitlements to different types of services, the main financial responsibilities and principal providers. The refugees are identified as a distinct subpopulation, with its own basic health services financed and delivered directly by UNRWA. Many of the refugee population also make use of government services although the exact figures are not known. An important component missing in Table A 10.5 is the contribution from the private corporations and employers to health financing. For example, the GHI scheme does not require direct contributions from the employers. Data are also not available on the extent to which private corporations contribute to their employees' health benefits.

Table A 10.5: Structure of the Health Systems: Entitlements, Financial Responsibilities and Principal Providers in West Bank and Gaza, 1996

Type of Services	Entitlement /[1]	Direct Financial Responsibility (principal payers)	Principal Providers
All Population: Preventive Care /Public Health	All citizens/[1]	Government	Government, NGOs
Early Child Care (0 - 3 Years); Antenatal and Postnatal Care	All citizens	Government	Government, NGOs
Primary Curative Care	GHI holders (50 percent of households)	Government (budget, GHI), Households (fees)	Government health services, private practitioners, NGOs
Secondary and Tertiary Care	GHI holders, police and security forces ?	Government(budget, GHI), and households (premium, co-payments or fees for service)/[2]	Government, NGO/ private providers, overseas providers
Rehabilitation	All citizens	Government, NGOs	NGO rehabilitation clinics
Mental Health	All citizens	Government	Government
Dental	Selective services covered by government health service	Government, households (fees for service)	Government PHC centers, private practitioners
Refugee Population:[3] Primary Care	Free care for refugees	UNRWA (external assistance)	UNRWA health centers
Secondary Care	A limited number of cases approved for referral	UNRWA and households (cost-sharing)	Subcontracted hospitals (NGO, overseas), one UNRWA hospital

1. "Entitlement" refers to those services for which the citizens of WBG are, in principle, guaranteed some level of public financing: it is not equivalent to actual access to services, since that depends on the actual availability of government services in the area.
2. Social welfare cases have health insurance premiums paid by the government.
3. As noted in the text, the refugee population also have access to all of the government services if they participate in the GHI plan.
Source: Ministry of Health.

Table A 10.6 shows the relative capacities and activities of the hospitals in the three major subsectors. The government sector has become by far the largest provider of hospital services, and is expected to expand its capacity by as much as 35 percent over the next five years according to the current public investment plan. These investments will also increase the capacities in the government hospital services toward tertiary care services. There is some expected growth in the private/NGO sector, mainly through the building of private hospitals in West Bank and one at least one NGO (Palestine Red Crescent Society) hospital. UNRWA will continue to maintain its focus on basic primary care services. However, the new 230 bed European hospital in Khan Younis, will be managed initially by UNRWA, although its management is expected to be transferred to the MOH at an unspecified date in the future.

Table A 10.6: Distribution of Acute Care Hospital Beds and Discharges by Sector, 1996

Sector	Beds		Discharges	
	Number	Percent	Number	Percent
Ministry of Health	1,479	71	155,763	78
NGOs / Private	563	27	38,936	20
UNRWA	38	2	3,933	2
TOTAL	2,080	100	198,632	100

Source: Compiled from the data provided by MOH, Nablus and Gaza City; and UNRWA, 1997. These figures exclude: hospitals in East Jerusalem and psychiatric and rehabilitation hospitals that provide long-term care.

The MOH and UNRWA are the main providers of primary health care services in the WBG. although private practitioners working individually or through private/NGO clinics probably provide a significant share of first-contact physician services. Table A 10.7 summarizes the utilization rates of ambulatory services by different sectors. The number of visits to MOH facilities and NGO hospitals is based on actual recorded visits obtained from MOH database; the figure for UNRWA is an extrapolation from the 1995 data and the number for private practitioners is based on author's estimates. Although the number of visits to private practitioners is only an indicative figure, it underscores the importance of private physicians.

Table A 10.7: Distribution of Ambulatory and Primary Care Services by Sector, 1996

Sector	No. of Visits /a	Percent of total visits	Visits per Person
Total	**8,808,000**	**100**	**3.9**
Ministry of Health, Total	3,499,577	40	1.5
West Bank MOH Hospitals	530,431		
West Bank Public Health Facilities	1,507,732		
Gaza Strip MOH Hospitals	230,609		
Gaza Strip Public Health Facilities	1,230,805		
NGO Hospitals	103,055	1	0.05
UNRWA Health Services /b	2,500,000	28	1.9 /c
Private Practitioners /d	2,736,000	31	1.2

a. "Visits" include first time and repeat visits.
b. UNRWA figure is based on the extrapolation of 1995 data to 1996 using population growth rates (see Annex 11 for details).
c. Based on the refugee population only.
d. The number of visits to private practitioners is based on author's estimation, and should be treated as only indicative figures (see Annex 11 for details).
Sources: For MOH facilities and NGO hospitals, based on data provided by MOH, Nablus and Gaza City, 1997; for UNRWA health services, based on projections from 1995 figures in UNRWA Annual Report of the Department of Health, 1995; for private practitioners, author's estimates, see Annex Table 11.1.

HEALTH FINANCING IN WEST BANK AND GAZA

Government Sector

Financing and organizational structure. The MOH's present financing and organizational structure can be described as a hybrid between a social insurance system and an integrated health system based on general tax revenues. While the MOH exercises direct financial and administrative control over the government health providers, it functions as a third-party payer in respect to the overseas referral cases. With the expansion of the private providers in recent years, the MOH has also begun to purchase services from local private health care providers, albeit on a very limited basis. But despite this expansion in the purchasing role of the MOH, the GHI scheme has not yet evolved beyond its basic function as an earmarked tax collection mechanism to supplement the MOH budget. Other essential features of an insurance / purchasing agency, such as the designing, costing and evaluating the benefits packages for the insured population, the development of appropriate provider payment systems and contracting mechanisms with various providers, and fund management, have yet to be fully developed. This is not surprising given that the MOH's "purchasing" functions are circumscribed by the administrative procedures and regulation of the central government, and MOH exercises little financial autonomy over the GHI revenues.

International experience shows that universal coverage can be achieved either through a payroll-tax based social insurance system or through general tax-based health service system. However, no country relies exclusively on payroll tax alone to finance their health system: in the industrialized countries, social health insurance funds are supplemented in varying degrees by general revenues as a means of redistributing resources between different income groups. Developing countries tend to rely on general revenues for other reasons. Because of the limited number of the workforce in the formal wage-earning sector and the limited revenue collection capacity of governments, most middle income countries face difficulties in expanding the social insurance coverage. As a result, even in those countries where the social insurance system is relatively well-established, governments continue to rely on general revenues to supplement their social insurance receipts. Within the Middle East and North Africa (MENA) region Algeria derives about one third of health financing from social insurance receipts, the highest in the region. In the rest of the MENA region social insurance contributions account between 0 to 20 percent of the total health revenues. Against these statistics, the proportion of revenues derived from the GHI premium in the WBG (around 10 percent) appear to be fairly typical for its level of income and development.

Sources of revenues. In 1996 about 27 percent of revenues were collected from the GHI premium (including transfers from the Israeli Government for the insurance premium deducted from the Palestinian workers in Israel), 10 percent from copayments and fees collected by the health facilities, and the remaining 63 percent from general tax revenues.

Latest data on the actual receipts from insurance premium payments for the first half of 1997 show a significant increase over the previous year's first half. If this first half 1997 figure is used to project the revenues for the remainder of the year, the total MOH revenues for 1997 would increase by over 20 percent the 1996 level. This optimistic estimation assumes that there will be no closures or other economic disturbances in the remainder of 1997. The actual revenue for 1997 will probably fall somewhat below this projection.

Although enrollment rates have been expanding steadily over the last two years, a commensurate increase in revenues from the GHI sources has not been achieved. Table A 10.8 shows the average annual contribution rate per household for various categories of GHI beneficiaries. Except in the category of Group Contracts, the average household contribution rates have fallen between 1995 and 1996. The contribution rates among the voluntary participants (individual and group contracts) are only about half as much as the contribution level of the compulsory groups. These lower rates probably reflect not only the lower basic premium rate but a lower collection rate, since voluntary contributions are more difficult to verify and enforce.

About 10 percent of MOH revenues are derived from copayments, licensing fees and other fees collected by the health facilities. Copayments for drugs and diagnostic tests are collected in the form of "stamps", and these stamps give an indication of the level of service utilization by the insured population. As shown in Table 9 in 1996 insured households on average spent $19 per year on copayments. Households in Gaza Strip appear to make more frequent use of government health services than in West Bank, possibly a reflection of the fact that there are fewer alternative (NGO or private) providers in Gaza Strip than in West Bank. From the changes in copayments between 1995 and 1996, it can be inferred that the service utilization rates per household went up in Gaza Strip, but remained nearly constant in West Bank.

Table A 10.8: Average Annual Contributions per Household to Government Health Insurance Premium, 1995-96
(US$ at official exchange rate)

	1995	1996
West Bank and Gaza		
Voluntary	153	117
Group Contracts	81	133
Compulsory	256	246
Workers in Israel	248	218
Social Welfare Group	0	0
West Bank		
Voluntary	187	143
Group Contracts	136	167
Compulsory	266	239
Workers in Israel	163	177
Social Welfare Group	0	0
Gaza Strip		
Voluntary	123	84
Group Contracts	22	83
Compulsory	236	251
Workers in Israel	378	272
Social Welfare Group	0	0

Source: Calculated from data provided by MOH, Gaza City, 1997.

Table A 10.9: Average Annual Household Contributions in the Form of Stamps (Copayment) for Drugs and Diagnostic Services
(in US$ at official exchange rate)

	1995	1996
West Bank and Gaza	18	19
West Bank	15	14
Gaza Strip	21	26

Source: Calculated from data provided by the Health Insurance Department, Gaza City, MOH, 1997.

**Table A 10.10: Estimated Levels of Subsidies Per Insured Household, 1996
(in US$, official exchange rate)**

	Average per insured household			
	Expenditure on Hospitalization	Insurance Contribution	Copayments (stamps)	Subsidy for Hospitalization
West Bank and Gaza	333	176	19	138
West Bank	295	168	14	113
Gaza Strip	386	181	26	179

Source: Author's estimates. See Annex 17 for details.

Table A 10.10 compares the estimated expenditures on hospitalization with average household contribution rates. If all insured households contributed US$333 per year, then the premium contribution would cover the entire cost of hospitalization (including overseas treatment). At the present contribution rates, however, a dollar of contribution from the GHI participant is matched by about 80 cents of contribution from the general revenues towards the cost of hospitalization for all insured population. These figures do not include the costs of other services provided by the government, such as preventive care and public health programs which do not require insurance coverage and are therefore covered in its entirety by taxation.

The sources of revenues by different categories of GHI holders for 1996 are: compulsory (35 percent); workers in Israel (26 percent); voluntary - individual (13 percent); group contracts (12 percent); and copayments (stamps) (12 percent). Contributions from the workers in Israel tend to fluctuate during periods of uncertainties in the job market in Israel. Although the enrollment rates have expanded significantly for those on Group Contracts, their total contributions have been relatively small due to the very low premiums collected from this group. In fact, the total contributions from the voluntary participants have actually declined in the past year.

The unemployed and hardship cases are charged a minimum premium of NIS 40 per month for GHI coverage. The Ministry of Social Welfare, in principle, covers the premium cost (equivalent to about $150 per year) for household who qualify as social welfare cases. In 1996 the Ministry of Social Welfare would have contributed around US$ 5.3 million, or about 16 percent of the total GHI contributions, for about 35,000 households who were registered as social welfare cases. Presumably this amount would have been included in the budget allocation from the Treasury to the MOH, but this budget transfer is not formally recorded as an expenditure item for the Ministry of Social Welfare and a revenue item for the MOH.

Members of the Police Force contribute 2.5 percent of their base salary for medical care[59]. As in the case of the social welfare group, their contributions do not appear specifically as revenues for the GHI. A separate extrabudgetary account exists for financing the medical services for the Police Force. It is unclear whether all their contributions are allocated to a separate medical service account for the Police Force or to the MOH budget.

Enrollment and eligibility. The entire Palestinian population in the WBG is eligible for the GHI scheme, although there appears to be some questions regarding the eligibility of the overseas Palestinians. Enrollment in GHI grew from 20 percent of the total WBG population in 1993 under the Israeli Civil Administration, to over 35 percent in June 1997. The latest figures from the first half of 1997 indicate an accelerating growth in the enrollment rate.

---

[59] The GHI is covering about 25,000 households (average 5.2 persons per household) of the Police Force.

A number of critical changes introduced by the government on the GHI scheme have supported this rapid expansion in enrollment.

- The lowering the monthly premium rates from NIS 110 per month under the Civil Administration to variable rates of 5 percent of monthly wage or NIS 75 maximum has made the scheme more affordable to a larger segment of the population.

- For an additional NIS 15 per month, the first two dependents of the head of the household can be included in the GHI scheme (then for an additional NIS 35 per month additional dependents may be insured). This generous policy offers an added incentive to enroll in the scheme, particularly for families with ailing elderly parents. Since most Palestinian families retain an extended family structure, the policy has probably helped to bring a significant number of the elderly population under the GHI scheme, but has also contributed to a major escalation in cost of care. Data on the actual number and age of dependents under the GHI scheme are not available to confirm these trends[60].

- The introduction of the Group Contract scheme encourages employer groups and associations to purchase health insurance coverage for their employees or members at a discounted rate. This category has shown the highest expansion in enrollment in the last two years, but because of the very low premium rates their overall level of contribution has been low.

The number of households who enrolled voluntarily in the GHI, either as individuals or as members of the group contracts, more than tripled between 1993 and 1997. Group contracts are actively promoted by the MOH and are showing a strong growth in enrollment in 1997, but voluntary enrollment by individuals appears to have peaked in 1996. The number of workers in Israel has been growing relatively more slowly than the rest of the enrollees. Their contributions stop during border closures. Social welfare cases accounted for 20 percent of total GHI holders in 1996.

Data are not available on the composition and characteristics of the uninsured population. The existing policy of the voluntary participation in the GHI probably leads to some form of selection bias. The uninsured group probably includes the well-to-do households, many of whom have their own private insurance coverage, and the young and relatively healthy households who are at a low risk of falling ill. There is no waiting period to access primary care and a two months waiting period for hospitalization (though patients would have to pay 50 percent of annual contribution and 25 percent of hospital costs)[61]; in emergency cases patients are able to access overseas treatment upon payment of a full year's premium. This flexible and relatively easy enrollment requirements give households an incentive to stay out of the insurance until they are compelled to join when a member of the household falls ill.

Population with the refugee status are eligible for free basic health services from UNRWA, but many also enroll in the GHI scheme although they are likely to be government employees who are required to enroll. This cross-over is probably encouraged by the overcrowding and limited services available at UNRWA health facilities. Most UNRWA health

---

[60] The most recent estimate of the average family size in Gaza Strip is 6 persons (the MOH, 1997).

[61] Insured patients, after the waiting period, pay 25 percent of hospital costs excluding certain conditions including heart disease, kidney disease and cancers.

facilities are located within the camps and are used mainly by the residents in these camps. Refugees who reside outside of the camps (mainly in West Bank) are more likely to make use of the government facilities.

Details on the premiums, copayment rates and benefits of the GHI scheme are discussed in Annex 5.

Figure A 10.2: Enrollment Patterns in Government Health Insurance, 1993-96

A. Number of Households Enrolled

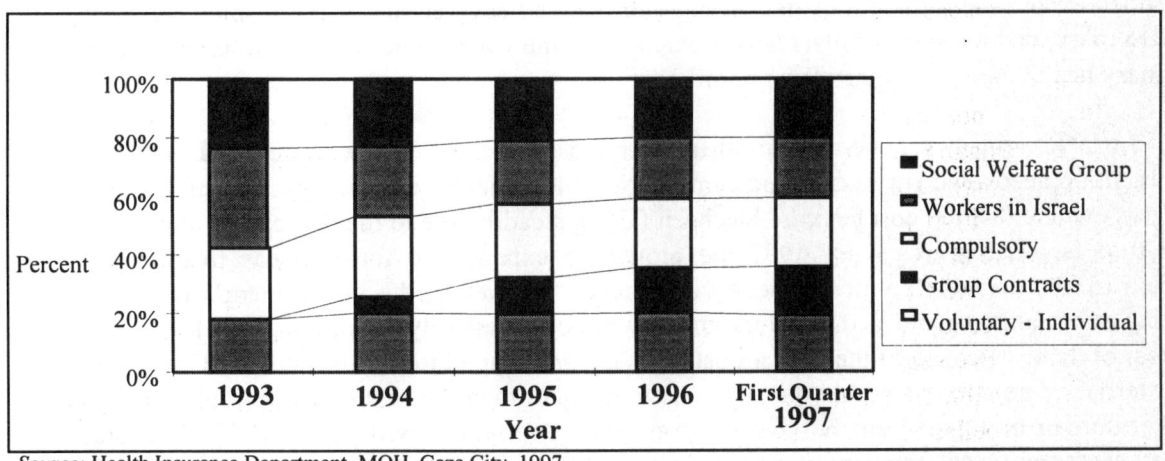

B. Percent Distribution, 1993-97

Source: Health Insurance Department, MOH, Gaza City, 1997.

Budgeting and resource allocation process. MOH follows the standard centralized budgeting process typical of a traditional public administration, which emphasizes control over efficiency. Ministry of Finance (MOF) transfers monthly advance to the MOH's current expenditure account based on a ceiling established by the annual budget, and MOH must contain expenditures to within the limits set for each line-item. Revenues from the insurance premium payments and copayments collected at points of service are also transferred directly to the MOF accounts, and the MOH does not have direct access to these funds. The MOH, in turn, centrally manages the financing and procurement requirements for all of the public health facilities (hospitals, primary health care centers) under its administration. Financial management is, therefore, almost nonexistent at the facilities level, since all the necessary information and authority for making financial decisions are held at the central ministry level.

Expenditure Patterns. Figure A 10.3 presents the MOH expenditure pattern by types of inputs for 1993-97. Between 1995-97 drug expenditures accounted for the fastest growing component in the MOH's expenditure item. Serious attention is needed to introduce drug policies and reforms that will reverse the rise in drug consumption rate. The projected decline in the salary component is another source of concern. MOH salary increases have been held down for number of years already, and are fueling considerable dissatisfaction among the MOH staff. Any further deterioration in the wage rate will likely have serious consequences on the quality of care and may lead to labor unrest.

In the government hospitals in West Bank, salaries accounted for 42 percent of total expenditures in 1996. By comparison, in the UNRWA hospital in Qalqilya, salaries accounted for about 76 percent of total hospital expenditure. Some of this difference can be attributed to the fact that MOH hospitals manage more complex cases than the UNRWA hospital, and are therefore likely to have higher drug costs. However, a significant portion of the difference could also be due to wage differentials. In the MOH primary health care services, salaries accounted for about 39 percent of the total in 1996.

Figure A 10.4 shows the MOH expenditure for different levels of health care in West Bank. Similar data for Gaza Strip were not available at this time. Secondary and tertiary care services accounted for nearly two thirds of the total MOH expenditure in West Bank while primary health care ("public health services") accounted for less than a quarter of the total. In the medium-term the expenditures on overseas treatment are expected to decline as increasing number of tertiary cases become admitted to the local private or government hospitals. Under the planned expansion of the public delivery system with a heavy emphasis on hospital capacity, the share of expenditure on hospitals will probably become even higher relative to expenditures on primary health care (see Annex 9 for details).

In 1996, around 3.7 percent of all inpatient cases in the WBG were referred overseas, and this group accounted for over 16 percent of total MOH health expenditure. From Table A 10.11 it is evident that the cost per case has been falling steadily due to the decreasing number of referrals to Israeli hospitals. By 1997 the growth in expenditure for overseas treatment is projected to be contained to the previous year's level. However, the government's policy of replacing overseas treatment with local treatment will not necessarily result in a reduction in the total cost of care. Because of the higher cost of living and wage rates within the WBG, the unit cost of tertiary care services within the WBG will be higher than the cost of comparable services in either Jordan or Egypt. In the coming years the government will face a difficult choice between promoting local capacity or on saving costs by purchasing services from the relatively less expensive overseas providers.

Figure A 10.3: Ministry of Health - Expenditures Patterns, 1993-97

A. In Thousands of US$

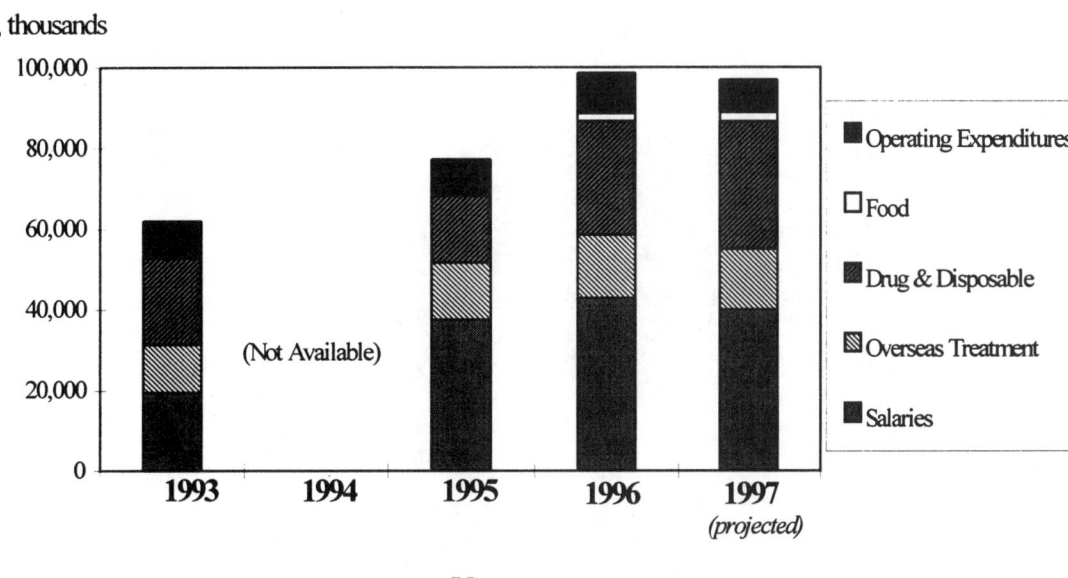

B. Percent Distribution

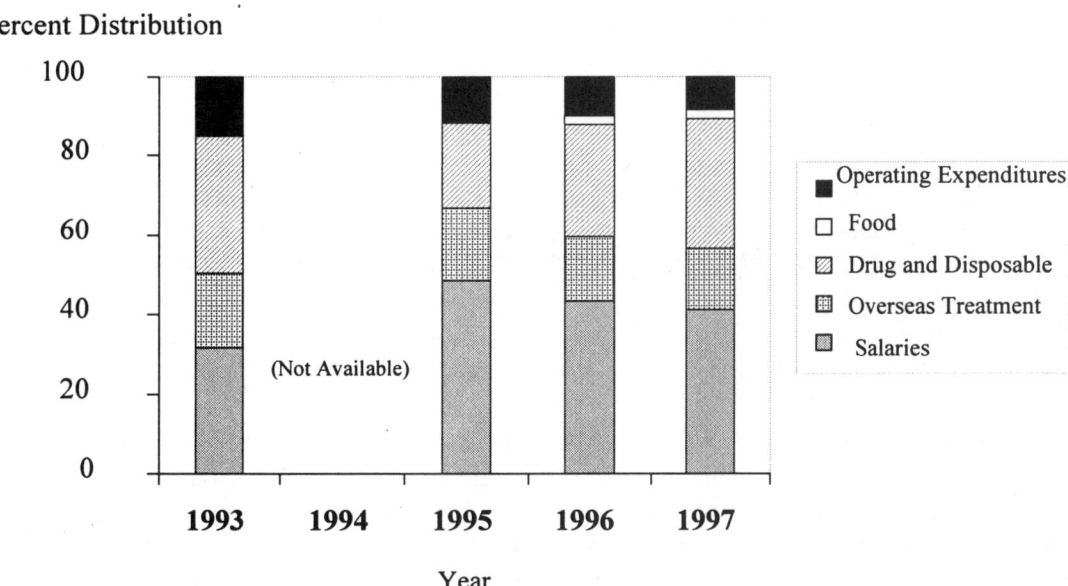

**Figure A 10.4: Ministry of Health Expenditures
by Levels of Health Care in West Bank, 1996**

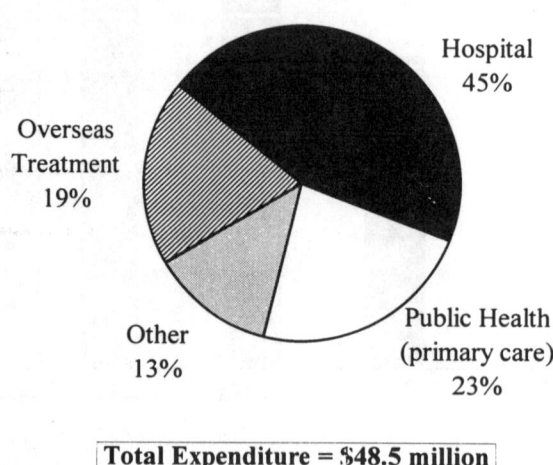

Total Expenditure = $48.5 million

Source: Based on (a) 1996 expenditure data on hospitals and public health care services from the Finance Department, the MOH, Nablus, and (b) data on expenditure for overseas treatment for West Bank provided by the MOH, Gaza City.

Table A 10.11: Overseas Referral - Number of Cases, Average Cost per Case, 1993-96

	1993	1995	1996
West Bank and Gaza			
Number of Cases Referred	2,462	5,804	6,725
Total Cost (US$, thousands)	11,702	14,114	15,707
Average Cost per Case (US$)	4,753	2,432	2,294

Source: Based on data provided by the MOH, Gaza City, 1997.

EXTERNAL ASSISTANCE

External assistance continues to be a significant source of revenues for the health sector in the WBG. They account for most of the capital and development costs for both the public and the NGO sectors. Table A 10.5 and Table A 10.12 present the breakdown of external assistance by types of assistance. Technical assistance or public investment which accounted for about 80 percent of total external assistance between 1994 and 1996.   Transitional budget support amounted to less than 5 percent of the total over the same period.

According to the latest public investment priorities submitted by the MOH, the proposed investments in the health sector over the next five years amount to around US$275 million (see Table A 10.13), of which 80 percent will be directed towards the expansion of hospital sector. MOH will seek external assistance to finance most of the proposed investment programs.

Table A 10.12: External Assistance - Disbursements by Type of Assistance, 1994-97

Type of Assistance	Disbursements (percent)			
	1994	1995	1996	1997 (first quarter)
Technical Assistance	40	61	21	78
Public Investment	38	17	60	9
Equipment	8	17	2	0
In-kind Contribution	10	1	12	0
Transitional Budget Support	3	4	6	13
Others	1	1	0	0
Total	100	100	100	100
Total Amount in US$, Millions	33.3	32.7	43.4	6.5

Source: MOPIC, 1997

Figure A 10.5: External Assistance, 1994 -first quarter 1997

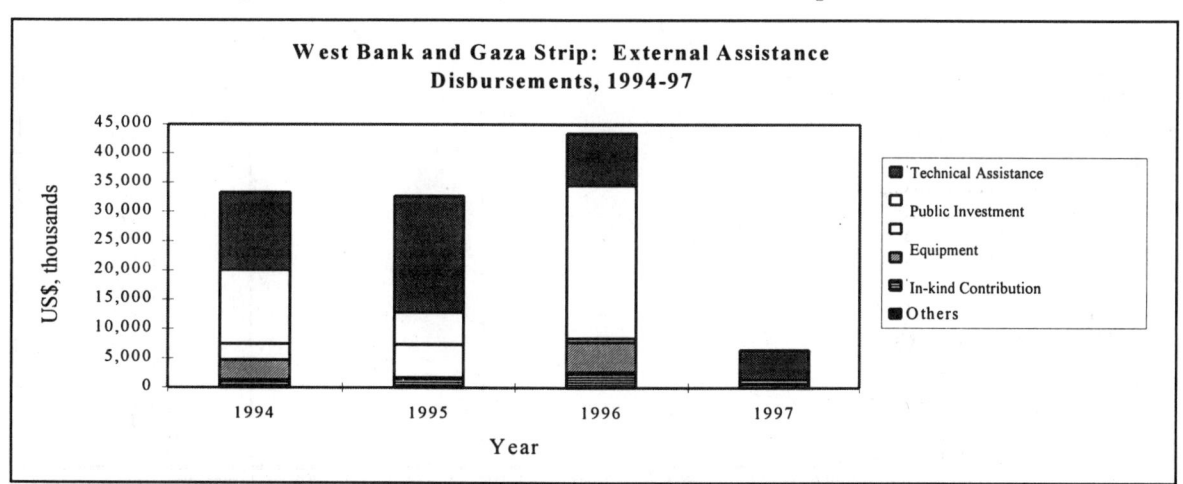

Source: Ministry of Planning and International Cooperation (MOPIC), 1997.

**Table A 10.13: Proposed Public Investment Plan for External Assistance, 1997-2002
(in millions of US$, at constant 1997 price)**

	1997	1998	1999	2000	2001	2002	Total
Hospital Sector /[1]	35.1	35.1	35.1	35.1	35.1	35.1	211.7
Primary Health Care	11.1	8.5	8.5	6.9	4.2	4	43.1
Others /[2]	2.0	2.0	2.0	2.0	2.0	2.0	12.1
Total	48.2	45.6	45.6	44.0	41.3	41.1	265.6

1. The exact phasing of investments for "hospital" and "others" category are not known. Hence, these investments have been equally distributed over the 6 year period.
2. "Others" include investments in nursing school, central stores, public health laboratory and central maintenance workshop.
Source: Compiled from data provided by the MOH, June 1997. See Annex 9 for details.

UNRWA

In the medium-term UNRWA will continue to provide basic health services mainly to the refugee population living in camps. Table A 10.14 provides a detailed breakdown of UNRWA expenditures on health services in the WBG in 1995-96 . Although the main thrust of UNRWA's services are in the area of basic primary health care, the breakdown in expenditures shows that 20 percent of the total budget was spent on secondary hospitalization in 1996. Except for the Qalqilya hospital (38 beds), most of the inpatient care is purchased through subcontracts or direct reimbursements with the NGO hospitals. Drugs and supplies accounted for 11 percent of the expenditure, salaries 38 percent, operating expenditures for primary care 20 percent, and capital spending 10 percent.

Table A 10.14: UNRWA Expenditure on Health Services, 1995-96
(US$, thousands)

	1995	1996
West Bank		
Primary Health Care (excluding staff costs)	Not Available	3,298
Secondary Health Care	N/A	
- Reimbursements	N/A	606
- Contracts	N/A	1,822
- Qalqilya Hospital (38 beds)	N/A	1,012
Salaries	N/A	3,789
Drugs and Disposables	N/A	874
Capital Spending (equipment and construction)	N/A	1,062
Gaza Strip		
Recurrent Costs	2,028	1,569
Secondary Health Care		
Subcontracts	1,570	1,315
Salaries	5,346	5,009
Drugs and Other Supplies	1,306	1,682
Health Education Program	79	8
Capital Spending (equipment and construction)	2,422	1,134
West Bank and Gaza Total		**23,180**

Source: Compiled from data provided by the UNRWA Administrative Offices in Gaza City and East Jerusalem, 1997. .

NONGOVERNMENTAL ORGANIZATIONS

Barghouti and Lennock (1997) have already described the NGO sector in some detail. Although very little information is available on the recent financial status of the NGOs, it appears that since 1994 there seems to have been a steep decline in the level of donations accruing to the NGO sector. This has led to a number of closures and reduction in services provided by the NGOs.   Nonetheless, NGO hospitals and clinics still account for over a quarter of the acute care beds and provide services for about a fifth of all patients in the WBG (see Table A 10.6, above). Recently, the MOH has begun to refer some of its patients to NGO clinics (e.g. the Patient Friendship Hospitals) for secondary care, but the flow of funds from government health insurance to NGO providers remains fairly restricted.

With the decline in donations from charitable sources, many of the NGOs are relying increasingly to revenues from patient fees, some of which are quite high. A number of facilities are also being bought out or are entering into a joint venture with private investors (e.g. St. Lukes in Nablus which is jointly developing a cardiac unit with Arabcare Medical Services; and the ophthalmic hospital in Bethlehem has been sold to Medlab). As a result, the distinction between an NGO and private, for-profit, organization is becoming blurred. In the absence of a well-defined legal framework for the governance for the NGO sector, the exact mandates and roles of the NGOs remain unclear.

PRIVATE SECTOR

Household Expenditure Patterns

Direct household expenditure on medical care accounted for about 40 percent of the total health expenditure in WBG. According to the Palestinian Expenditure and Consumption Survey (October 1995 to September 1996) conducted by the Palestinian Central Bureau of Statistics, average monthly household expenditure was US$828, of which US$29, or 3.5 percent of the total, was spent on medical care and health insurance premiums (see Table A 10.15). Households in West Bank spent higher percentage of household resources on medical care, and households which are better off also spent a higher percentage of resources on medical care.

Table A 10.15 also includes the data on the average consumption of tobacco as a percentage of total household expenditure in the WBG. Tobacco consumption accounted for 4 percent of the total household consumption, compared with 3.5 percent on medical care. In other words, most households spend more on the purchase of tobacco than on medical services. This household behavior presents a significant challenge to the public health community.

Table A 10.15: Monthly Household Expenditure on Medical Care, 1996

Category	Monthly Household Expenditures in US$		Percent of Household Expenditure	
	Total	Medical Care[a]	Medical Care	Tobacco Consumption
West Bank and Gaza	828	29	3.5	4.0
West Bank	879	33	3.7	4.0
Gaza Strip	703	19	2.8	3.9
Level of Living [b]				
Worse-off	639	20	3.1	3.8
Middle	835	30	3.5	4.6
Well-off	1,172	44	3.8	3.3

a. Includes household expenditures on health insurance premiums.
b. Worse off = households with food consumption greater than 45 percent of total; middle = 30 percent to 44 percent of total consumption; Better off = less than 30 percent of total consumption.
Source: Palestinian Central Bureau of Statistics Expenditure and Consumption Survey, Ramallah, West Bank, 1996.

Table A 10.16 shows a more detailed breakdown of household expenditures by different categories of medical services and goods. Purchase of drugs account for almost 40 percent of the total household expenditure on medical care, followed by health insurance premiums (19 percent) and physician services (18 percent). Household expenditures in Gaza Strip was only about 60 percent of the West Bank expenditure, probably reflecting the lower average income level in Gaza Strip (approximately half of West Bank).

A notable difference exists between West Bank and Gaza Strip in the level of health insurance coverage and out-of-pocket expenditure on hospitalization. Households in West Bank spent around $7 per capita on health insurance premium whereas households in Gaza Strip spent over $10 per capita, despite the lower income levels. On the other hand, households in Gaza Strip spent less than a dollar per capita on hospitalization compared to nearly $11 in the West Bank. This expenditure pattern suggests that in Gaza Strip households are more likely to rely on government hospitals where they receive free care if they are insured, whereas more households in West Bank opt to go to NGO / private hospitals and clinics where they must pay fairly substantial fees for hospitalization. This points to important differences in the utilization of medical services between households in the West Bank and Gaza Strip.

Table A 10.16: Household Expenditure on Medical Care, 1996 - Annual per capita expenditure, in US$

Categories of Health Expenditure	West Bank	Gaza Strip	West Bank and Gaza	Percent Distribution
Physician Services	12.62	6.33	9.26	18
Hospitalization	10.78	0.78	4.81	9
Dental Care	4.70	1.32	2.75	5
Drugs	25.83	15.62	20.74	39
Diagnostic Tests, X-Rays	3.59	1.55	2.47	5
Other Medical Expenses	1.87	2.83	2.64	5
Health Insurance Premium	7.04	10.80	10.03	19
Total	66.43	39.22	52.70	100

Source: Calculated from data from the Palestinian Expenditure and Consumption Survey, Palestinian Central Bureau of Statistics, unpublished report, Ramallah, West Bank, 1997.

Box 1: Consultation Fees for Private Medical Practitioners

The following figures, provided by the Palestinian Medical Association, Ramallah, West Bank, represent the recommended rates to be charged by private practitioners in the West Bank and Gaza Strip. The fees are based on the rates established by the Jordanian Medical Association and have not been updated for some years. All figures are in New Israeli Shekels (NIS).

	Minimum	Maximum
1. First visits		
General Practitioners	15	50
Specialists	25	50
2. Repeat visits		
(within two weeks, for the same diagnosis):	Free of charge	
3. Home visits		
- Day visit		
General Practitioner	30	50
Specialist	50	100
- Night visit		
General Practitioner	45	75
Specialist	75	150
- Night visit at physician's home		
General Practitioner	30	50
Specialist	50	100

Private Practitioners

Very little information is available on the number of activities of the private practitioners, but they probably account for a significant percentage of physician visits in the WBG (see Table A 10.7). Private practitioners receive fees for services from the patients and through a contractual arrangements with private insurance companies. After the purchase of drugs and insurance premiums, payments for physician services account for the next largest expenditure item of household spending on medical care. Data are also not available for fees charged for each visit to a private physician, but the Palestinian Medical Association in the West

Bank has a recommended fee schedule for physician visits (see Box 1 below). Recommended fees range from NIS 30 to 50 for general practitioners and specialists and NIS 50 to 100 for specialists visits during the day.

In the West Bank some private practitioners are organized into a group practice or operate out of NGO or private clinics, often on contractual basis. The MOH does not have any contractual or reimbursement procedures with regard to the private practitioners. Many of the public doctors are known to have private practice during their off-duty hours, and this creates a variety of problems related to conflict of interests between the private and public sectors.

Private Insurance

Very little information is available on the coverage and scope of private health insurance in the WBG. Barghouti and Lennock (1997) provide information on the two major private insurance companies, the Arab Insurance Company and Al-Mushriq Company. In 1996 these companies charged about US$734 per year for a family of four (compared with around US$ 130-250 for GHI premiums), and excluded applicants with pre-existing conditions. Table A 10.17 shows a profile of another small private insurance company, Trust International, which began offering private health insurance plans in April 1996. These private companies cover only a very small fraction (2.7 percent) of the total population.

Private insurance companies appear to be encountering problems typical of a nascent health insurance market. The presence of a relatively cheap government health insurance also acts as a deterrent to the development of private health insurance schemes. The Trust International, faced difficulties in attracting sufficient number of households, did not initially exclude the elderly or those with pre-existing conditions. Those who enrolled were probably self-selected for households most likely to have medical expenses, and consequently the medical expenditures for 1996 far exceeded their premium revenues. As in the case of the other insurance companies, from 1997, the Trust International has also begun to select out the high risk cases (e.g., exclusion of members over 65 years of age and those with pre-existing conditions).

Table A 10.17: Profile of a Private Health Insurance Plan (Trust International Company)

	May 1996 - April 1997	*May 1997 - April 1998*
Premium Rates	JD 230 per family of 4	JD 300/[a] per family of 4
	JD 40 per additional child	JD 50 for additional dependents
	JD 30 per parent, including those over 65 years of age	Excluded: dependents over 65 years of age
	--	JD 130 for single individual
Benefits	Access to all private sector providers	Access to all private sector providers
Eligibility	All members and dependents of the Federal Labor Union	Members of the Federal Labor Union and dependents, but excludes individuals over 65 years of age and those with pre-existing conditions

a. By way of comparison, a contribution rate of JD 300 per year is equivalent to about US$415 per year.
Source:: Interview with Ms. Rana Shunnar, Trust International, Ramallah, May 21, 1997.

Private Investors

Table A 10.18, below, summarizes the investment plans of two major private investors in the WBG. Most of these investments are in the area of high technology diagnostic services or in specialized hospital services. These investments amount to around US$ 40 million, or around 15 percent of the public investments being proposed for the WBG over the same period (see External Assistance, above).

Table A 10.18: Private Investments in West Bank and Gaza Health System

Description of Services and Facilities	Investment Amount, US$ million	Estimated Year of Completion
Arabcare Medical Services		
Surda Hospital, Ramallah - 100 Bed General Surgical Hospital	18.5	2000
Diagnostic Units, Gaza and Nablus	0.3	-
Ramallah Medical Center - Diagnostic Unit, Polyclinic and 20 Bed Surgery Ward	3.6	1997
Nablus Diagnostic Center - St. Lukes Hospital - Cardiac Unit	3.9	1997
Subtotal	26	
Medlab		
Bethlehem Hospital - Specialized Services, 68 Beds	-	1997?
Ramallah In-Vitro Fertilization Center	-	1996
Diagnostic Units, Nablus, Ramallah, Hebron And Gaza	-	
Subtotal	14.0	

Sources: Arabcare Medical Services, Ramallah, 1997; and Barghouti and Lennock, 1997.

AFFORDABILITY AND SUSTAINABILITY OF THE HEALTH FINANCING SYSTEM

As indicated in the preceding discussions, both the government and private investors are gearing up for a major expansion in health service capacity at a time when economic recession and growing unemployment rates are likely to lead to resource constraints at all levels of the economy. According to the latest current public investment plan, the MOH sector will expand its service capacity by 957 new beds (and 1,157 new beds if the EU Hospital is included under MOH management) and 96 new primary health care units by the year 2002. This could add about US$70 million in operating costs (at constant 1997 prices), or about 70 percent increase in real value over the current expenditure level. This translates to an increase in budget of 12 percent per year in real terms in the next five years just to cover the additional recurrent cost of the expanded services (see Annex 9 for details).

Table A 10.19: Ministry of Health - Projected Incremental Recurrent Cost of Expanded MOH Facilities, 1998-2002 (in US$ million, at constant 1997 price)

Year	1998	1999	2000	2001	2002
Hospitals	19.8	32.2	39.8	46.3	54.9
Primary Health Care Centers	6.8	9.8	12.2	13.7	15.1
Total Additional Recurrent Costs	26.7	42.0	52.0	61.0	69.9

Source: Estimated from investment data shown in Table A 10.13, above. The recurrent cost estimates were based on 25 percent of investment costs (excluding rehabilitation or renovation) for the hospital sector, and 40 percent of investment costs for PHC centers. See Annex 9 for an explanation of the assumptions and estimations used.

In addition, real cost increases will be expected to occur for other subcomponents of health services, including public health programs, medical education, and administration. A significant wage increase for the government health workers would also increase the overall expenditure level. Some cost savings will be possible from the rationalization of drug use. The overseas component will be substituted to some extent by services subcontracted or reimbursed from the new private providers, but this will not contribute to much cost savings due to the relatively high cost of running health services within the WBG. On the whole, MOH expenditure will likely increase at a rate significantly above 11 percent per year.

It is uncertain whether this rate of growth in expenditure can be sustained during a period of economic retrenchment. In order to cover the recurrent cost of the additional hospital and primary health care services, the government will need to increase revenues from GHI enrollment rate, for example, by about 15 percent per year for the next five years at a contribution rate of $250 per household (at constant 1997 price). Any shortfall below this level will have to be made up from taxation.

The proximity of Israel, with a per capita income and health expenditure at around ten times that of the WBG, has raised expectations on the part of the Palestinian population for a level of medical care and technology which might be difficult to sustain at their present income levels. For example, the number of MRIs per million population in the West Bank already exceeds that of UK and Canada - countries that spend between US$2,000 to US$3,000 per capita on health services, compared to US$120 per capita spent in Palestine. Maintaining and operating these high technology instruments is extremely costly irrespective of the volume of usage. Therefore they should only be introduced with the most judicious care.

Figure A 10.6: International Comparisons of Diagnostic Technology - MRIs

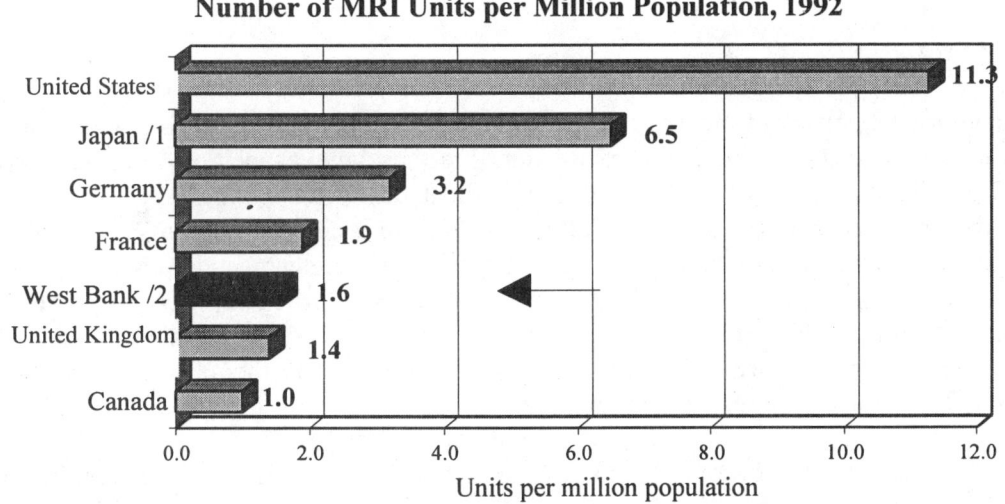

Number of MRI Units per Million Population, 1992

1. 1990 figure for Japan.
2. 1997 figure for West Bank.

Source: OECD Health Data Base, 1996 for figures on OECD countries. World Bank staff estimate for West Bank figure.

The MOH will need to re-evaluate the effectiveness of the current medical practices and choice of medical technology and drugs, cut down on the costly treatments that have a relatively low impact on health outcomes, and develop its own set of priorities more in keeping with a realistic assessment of its available resource. Overextending the system beyond its capacity to support itself will inevitably lead to underfinancing of services, which will quickly become manifest through deterioration in the quality of care, including labor unrest from underpaid and demoralized workers, public dissatisfaction with the poor services, and eventually deterioration in public support and declining willingness to pay for government services.

EFFICIENCY AND QUALITY OF CARE

This section identifies some of the major sources of inefficiencies in financing, investment strategies, utilization patterns and organization of health services.

Revenue Raising

In the short-term, there is limited scope for expanding the revenue stream of the government, but some room for improving the efficiency of the current GHI collection system exists. Some of the inefficiencies in revenue collection comes from: (i) the evasion of payments, especially by the voluntary contributors, (ii) the low ceiling on premiums which means those who have greater ability to pay contribute less to the system, and (iii) the lack of contributions from the employers, who are potentially a very important contributors to health financing. The voluntary nature of participation in the GHI also introduces selection bias which inevitably reduces the effectiveness of the risk-pooling function of the GHI scheme. The PA would also need to clarify policies regarding the contributions from the social welfare group (MOH estimates that the GHI program is owed about US$5 million in lieu of services offered to social welfare cases). Finally a better coordination between the GHI schemes and private insurance market could also increase the level of resources that could be mobilized from the private sector.

Investment Strategies

A significant portion of investments, both in the public and private sectors, is focused on the upgrading of medical technology and expansion of tertiary level capacities. Because this is a sector that entails major infusion of capital and is most costly to operate, any expansion of capacities requires particularly careful consideration. Rising incidence rates of cardiovascular diseases, diabetes and kidney diseases, injuries from auto accidents and burns, congenital diseases, complications during delivery all indicate the need for tertiary level care. However, a number of questions should be raised regarding the appropriateness of the number, the type and the organization of tertiary care services currently being proposed in the WBG. A number of potential sources of inefficiencies are identified below:

- As noted above, the 2 MRIs in the West Bank might already appear to be fairly high with respect to the size of the population, and raises fundamental questions about appropriateness of the medical technologies being introduced into the region.

- There is probably some duplication of tertiary care services being introduced in the government and private or NGO hospitals. These could be reduced through better intersectoral coordination and planning of services.

- For some of the tertiary care services, it could be more cost-effective to purchase from an overseas provider, particularly if the volume of demand is very low, instead of investing in local capacities; these policy options need to be evaluated in terms of cost and quality of care.

- Tertiary care services are being introduced through the upgrading or introduction of new units within the existing hospitals, most of which are very small (around 100 beds) by international standards. Small volume and turnover rates create enormous inefficiencies at the tertiary level. From the perspective of economy of scope, quality of care and staffing issues, the present strategy might require some rethinking.

- Because the GHI reimbursements are skewed towards the tertiary care services, the present payment system sends signals to the private investors to enter the market at the high technology end of the services. This might require further review to achieve a better balance the types of care being provided by the private sector.

The investments in both the public and private sector are heavily skewed towards the high technology curative services, while relatively small amounts are being proposed for preventive programs and services that could help to reduce the incidence of diseases and injuries that eventually require costly tertiary care services. For example, better traffic control could reduce road accidents, improvements in diet and decrease in tobacco smoking could reduce cardiovascular diseases; and better environmental regulation and occupational health could reduce incidence of burns and injuries at home and at workplace.

Utilization of Health Services

Hospital sector. From the available government statistics it is estimated that the inpatient admission rate in 1996 was around 9 percent of the population with an average length of stay of 3 days. This seems to be a somewhat high admission rate for a population in which less than 3 percent are above 65 years of age, although a more detailed study on the hospital utilization patterns and quality of care are needed to evaluate the appropriateness of hospital admissions. The very short length of stay raises a number of issues that require further analysis in terms of efficiency and quality of care. First, it suggests that some efficiency gain might be made by treating some of the hospital admissions in a day-care or outpatient basis. Secondly, it might indicate the likelihood of premature discharges to free up beds in some of the overcrowded government hospitals. There is some anecdotal evidence that this is indeed occurring in some hospitals. On the other hand, since most of the complex, tertiary cases are referred to overseas providers, the average length of stay would be expected to be relatively short in WBG hospitals.

A bed capacity of 0.9 beds per 1,000 population can accommodate a 9 percent admission rate at an average length of stay of three days, if all the beds are fully utilized at 80 percent occupancy rate (see Annex 10 for projected inpatient requirements). At present, there are about 2,300 acute care beds in the WBG[62], or around 1.0 bed per 1,000 population. If the overseas treatment cases are included, then the net effective bed capacity is around 1.1 bed per 1,000. The utilization rates are uneven among hospitals in different sectors as shown in Table A 10.20. Most of the government hospitals are operating at or above capacity, and overcrowding seems to be a problem at many of these hospitals: the turnover rates are very high and average length of stay in these hospitals is short. Patients are known to complain frequently about the poor attitude of the staff, which might due to overcrowding. Meanwhile, most NGO hospitals, especially the small NGO maternity clinics with average 10 beds, are operating below capacity. As discussed earlier, part of the low utilization rate at NGO hospitals can be attributed to a lack of insurance coverage for patients admitted to NGO hospitals. Expansion of insurance benefits to include the NGO hospitals could help to increase their utilization rates, and hence promote a more efficient use of available capacity.

---

[62] About 100 beds are added after the PA took over the responsibility.

Table A 10.20: Hospital Capacity and Utilization Pattern, 1996

	Share of Acute Bed Capacity (percent)	Size of Hospital/ Clinic (beds)	Bed Occupancy Rate (percent)	Average Length of Stay (days)
Government Hospitals				
West Bank	34	50 - 142	84	2.8
Gaza Strip	36	31 - 492	81	3.2
NGO Hospitals	22	10 - 88	64	3.1
NGO Maternity Clinics	6	10 - 12	24	1.2
UNRWA Qalqilya Hospital	2	38	114	2.8

Source: See Annex 7 for details on hospital capacity and utilization data.

By year 2002, it is estimated that there will be around 3,700 beds if all of the proposed investments in public and private hospitals are implemented as planned. This will be equivalent to about 1.3 beds per 1,000 population assuming an annual population growth rate of 4 percent over this period. To maintain this constant level of bed capacity at population growth rate of 4 percent, it will be necessary to expand the bed capacity by 100 new beds each year. At this capacity level, it would be theoretically possible to accommodate over 9 percent admission rate at an average length of stay of four days and 80 percent occupancy rate. This capacity level is probably more than sufficient to cover the needs of the current population. However, should the overall bed occupancy rate fall to 70 percent, then this bed capacity will accommodate only 8 percent admission rate, equivalent to a 13 percent decrease in effective capacity, while the fixed cost of running of the hospital remains the same. Thus, maintaining efficiency through full utilization of capacity has a major impact on the unit cost of hospital services.

Primary care / physician consultation pattern and payment system. Although a large number of primary care visits probably occur at the MOH primary health care (PHC) centers, many of these facilities appear to operate on very short or uncertain operating hours. This pattern appears to be more pronounced in the rural West Bank, where PHC facilities tend to be more widely dispersed and isolated from supervision and support compared to the PHC services in urban settings. It results in a relatively low utilization rate of the PHC facilities, and encourages patients to skip the primary level and go directly to emergency services at hospitals which are open 24 hours a day. Current MOH plans both to expand the number of PHC centers and to extend the operating hours will improve access to primary care services but it will require a significant increase in the staff hours to operate these centers. It is questionable whether this could be accomplished efficiently by increasing the staffing size of MOH workers, particularly when wage rates are considered very low. UNRWA health services, in contrast to the MOH services, have very high utilization rates, but tend to suffer from overcrowding, and patient consultation time is extremely short. Data on the quality and efficiency of services provided by the private practitioners are not available.

Inefficiencies in the Organization of the System

Microeconomic inefficiencies in the public sector. The MOH has generally followed a policy of expanding its own delivery system rather than through contracting or purchasing of services from the private or NGO sector. As a result, the health system will become increasingly dominated by a highly centralized and integrated health delivery system organized along the lines of the government bureaucratic system. A bureaucratic administrative structure is generally known to be ineffective at managing an complex modern health care financing and delivery systems. Line-item budgeting imposes an input-oriented rather than output oriented planning process; there is little scope for allowing money to follow the patient (i.e. allocation system based on utilization); and civil service regulations and administrative procedures impede the introduction of a more flexible, incentive system which rewards staff for good services, sanctions those that perform poorly and encourages initiatives and innovations. Thus, the expansion of such an organizational structure will exacerbate the inefficiencies in the system.

EQUITY AND ACCESS

With the expansion in the supply of delivery services within the WBG and in insurance coverage, access to care has generally improved for a large segment of the Palestinian population. But the system still falls far short of universal coverage, and recent economic trends will add to the difficulties in expanding coverage. The existing MOH financing system has established a number of features that result in a regressive revenue collection system. The relatively low ceiling on monthly insurance premium payments sets up a regressive system of revenue collection mechanism and allows a higher proportion of subsidies to accrue to the well-to-do. Moreover, after the social welfare group, the participants in the group contracts category receive the highest share of subsidies, even though they are probably more capable of contributing a higher premium rate.

The MOH will need better information on the characteristics of the insured and uninsured population in order to evaluate the redistributive effects of its financial policies. For example, at present there is no analysis available on the socio-economic profile of the uninsured population. The household consumption and expenditure survey conducted by the Central Statistical Bureau in 1996 should provide a good database for undertaking such an analysis. The effectiveness of the social welfare program in providing adequate health insurance coverage to the indigent families might also merit an independent study.

The voluntary nature of the GHI system presents a major challenge with regard to achieving equitable and universal access to health services. Systems that rely primarily on voluntary participation in health insurance tend to exhibit strong tendencies toward the segmentation of the population into groups with different risk profile. Often these groups are also correlated with different income levels and epidemiological profiles. Thus the growth of the private sector providers and insurance market increases the chances of a two-tiered system to develop. Consequently, most countries that have achieved universal coverage have relied on some form of public mandates, or through taxation or other forms of public financing to overcome this tendency toward fragmentation of the health financing market.

RECOMMENDATIONS: SHORT- TO MEDIUM-TERM ACTIONS

In view of recent economic downturn, there is a pressing need for the MOH to develop a coherent strategy for cost containment and rationalization of resources and, most importantly, to mobilize political and public support necessary for achieving many of the changes in the use and the delivery of services. Some of the priority areas for actions are suggested below.

Reevaluation of the public investment strategy

There is an urgent need to review the present public investment plan in terms of their affordability and sustainability, with greater attention to improving efficiency rather than on simply expanding capacity. As a start, the investment requirements should be based on a better understanding of expected demand and utilization of services rather than on a static normative standards of capacity (e.g. 2 beds per 1,000 population). Rapid technological changes, as well as the very different nature of epidemiological and demographic profiles, render this traditional mode of investment planning obsolete. An investment plan should include, at the very minimum, a specification of standards on buildings and equipment; projections of throughputs and estimations of fixed and variable costs at different levels of utilization; and the impact of public investments on the rest of the health systems (private, NGO and UNRWA).

Improving the efficiency of the GHI collection mechanism

Collection rates from the voluntary group are probably low because of relative difficulty in following up and enforcing regular payments on a voluntary basis: improvements in the information system, e.g. through computerized registration and payment records, could probably reduce some incidence of evasion among this group. Consideration should be given to raising the relatively low ceiling on the premium rates as well as mobilizing contributions from employers, for example through group contracts.

Defining a benefits package

Definition of a benefits package would help to identify the priority areas for public financing through investments, direct financing of services or reimbursements through the GHI scheme. The list of benefits covered by MOH (see Annex 5) as it is currently defined is too general to be effective as a means for rationalizing the health services. A more refined definition of benefits package could be developed, e.g. through negative lists (services excluded from public financing) or positive lists (services included in public financing). However, a definition of benefits package is not sufficient for rationalizing health services. For example, these benefits will need to be translated into provider payment systems and to appropriate medical protocols and procedures.

Rationalizing tertiary care services

Because of the complexity and the serious long-term cost implications of investments in the tertiary care sector, special attention will be needed to develop a coherent investment strategy in this sector. Priorities should be given to the introduction of the most effective (in medical terms), most appropriate (in terms of health outcomes and epidemiological profile of the population) and most cost-effective interventions. Consolidation of specialties within single hospitals rather than in providing multiple specialties in the many small hospitals. This exercise will need to be closely linked to a review of the medical technology as well as strategies for overseas referrals. There is some urgency in undertaking this review, since many of the investments in tertiary care services are already underway in both private and public sectors. Once these investments are made, it becomes extremely difficult as well as costly to reorganize the system. The government has two instruments for influencing the growth of tertiary care services in the private sector. The first is through direct regulation of capital investment and medical technology, e.g. through licensing or issuance of a certification of need in all sectors, public and private. The second is through its role as the purchaser of tertiary care services. MOH will need to reevaluate its current practice of reimbursing tertiary care services, and develop appropriate payment systems.

Improving complementarity between government and private/NGO hospital services

Expanding the benefits covered under the GHI scheme to include NGO and private providers would have the advantage of making a more efficient use of available resources as well as increasing the choice of providers for the patients. However, the MOH will need to overcome a number of constraints before expanding the purchasing function of the GHI scheme. First, the MOH's capacity to monitor the quality, efficiency and costs of the private or NGO hospitals is limited, and an appropriate provider payment system will need to be developed. Currently, all referrals outside of the government delivery system, both overseas and local, are approved on a case by case basis by the Medical Referral Committee: systems and procedures are not yet in place to manage and finance a high volume of cases treated outside of the government system. Secondly, a potential conflict of interest exists between the government doctors who also have part-time private practice in the NGO/private hospitals and clinics. The respective roles and responsibilities of the purchaser and providers should be clearly differentiated and regulated.

Improving the efficiency of primary health care services

As an alternative to direct expansion of the government-run primary health care system, MOH could explore the option of purchasing primary care services from other NGO clinics and private practitioners. Such a plan could provide a more flexible arrangement to meeting the needs of the population, make use of existing capacities in the other sectors, and improve the complementarity and coordination of primary care services among the different subsectors. One possible strategy would be contract qualified private practitioners to operate out of the government PHC centers. This will require the development of an appropriate physician payment system and a referral system which do not exist at the moment. Such a primary care system would provide a clearer delineation of the roles and responsibilities of the physician and, if proper designed, could circumvent the problems created by salaried public doctors engaging private practice on off-duty hours to augment their income. Another advantage is that it will also give the government greater flexibility in the management of PHC services, while introducing better regulation of the private practitioners. The ongoing program for training Family Doctors could help establish a basis for organizing the primary care physicians towards this direction.

Strengthening the referral system

A more stringent control of referral system at both the primary to secondary levels could go to some length at relieving the crowding and overuse of hospital emergency services. There is some scope for redesigning the copayment system to discourage the unnecessary use of hospital care and promote the appropriate use of primary care. Patients should be referred from a primary care physician to access hospital and specialist services. At the moment there is no financial penalty for patients who choose to skip this process, and many primary care patients enter the hospital system through the emergency unit. Any changes in the referral system would need to be accompanied by concurrent adjustments and improvements in the primary care services (e.g. better quality of care and longer operating hours in the government primary care clinics, and better incentives and training for the primary care physicians to function as gatekeepers).

Redefining the roles and functions of the MOH

The MOH will need to define and strengthen its role with respect to its (i) regulatory and policy-setting function, (ii) purchasing function; and (iii) service delivery / provider function.

To be more effective in its regulatory and policy-making functions, the Ministry will need to enhance its information system and data analysis capacity with respect to the entire health sector, including the private, NGO and UNRWA activities. In particular, the Ministry will need to improve its capacity to analyze the flow of funds (e.g. through the establishment of a national health accounts) in all sectors not limited to the public sector, and to assess the effectiveness of the subsidies and redistributive mechanisms in terms of ensuring equitable access to health services.

Regarding the insurance function of MOH, a number of immediate steps to strengthen the revenue collection capacity of the GHI were discussed above. In the medium-term, the purchasing function of the GHI will also need to be strengthened by developing its capacity to monitor and evaluate the cost, efficiency and quality of providers both within and outside of the government sector. This step will form a basis for future development of variety of provider payment systems (e.g., negotiating contracts, establishing tariffs, and estimating unit costs) that will be needed for the MOH to function as an effective purchaser of health services.

As for the MOH delivery systems, various measures are needed to strengthen the financial management at the facilities level. On a more immediate term, staff salaries and drug consumption are areas that require urgent attention. The implementation of the proposed essential drugs policies may help to contain expenditures on drugs. Some of the savings from the new drug policies could be applied towards increases in staff salaries, but such stop-gap measures will probably not suffice to deal with the problem of low wage rates. The government will need to undertake an in-depth review of the wage structure and staff deployment strategies to come up with viable solutions for the medium-term.

In the medium-term, the MOH will also need to develop a capacity for evaluating the performance of the public delivery system in terms of cost-effectiveness, efficiency and quality of service. This will include a development of management information systems and training and recruitment of managerial staff with strong finance and accounting background at the facilities level as well as the central level. These measures are a prerequisite to implementing a separation of provider and purchasing function within the MOH system. Concomitant changes in the legal status and governance structure of the delivery system (e.g. financial decentralization, managerial autonomy) would also need to be introduced in incremental steps.

Improving the complementarity between the private insurance market and public financing

For reasons outlined above, the government will need to be more proactive in directing the growth of the private insurance market. As a start, MOH will need information on the existing private insurance market, and identify areas where better complementarity could be achieved between the GHI and private insurance market. Selling a part of government health services to private insurers would be a controversial policy, but one in which MOH should be prepared to explore in the future. For example, if the proposed expansion in government delivery system creates excess capacity, it may become necessary to open these services to patients not covered under the GHI scheme.

Strengthening public education and mobilization of political support

Finally, the success of many of the proposed changes and improvements in the health systems will depend largely on the ability of the MOH to mobilize sufficient political and public support. The MOH will need to enhance its ability to communicate to its policies and programs, and to gather data and elicit responses from various constituencies (including the donor agencies). This might include the development of targeted public education programs, better marketing and customer relations program for the GHI scheme, and training and exposure of key policy-makers to a broad range of health systems and health policies and programs as practiced in other middle income and industrialized countries.

LONG-TERM OBJECTIVES: TOWARD A SYSTEM OF UNIVERSAL COVERAGE

The government has several option with regard to developing a system towards universal coverage. Three possible options are briefly outlined below.

National health service model (Integrated health system)

This approach most closely parallels the present investment strategy of the government, since it will involve the expansion of the public delivery system under the MOH rather than through the expansion in the purchasing function of the MOH. A major drawback of this type of health system is that it tends to expand an inefficient bureaucracy. At some point, therefore, the MOH would need to reform the delivery system to break away from the traditional administrative structure and by introducing greater separation between the provider and purchasing functions. Many countries with this form of health system are experimenting with the introduction of greater autonomy at the facility level. This will also entail the development of a provider payment system to guide the new relationship between the purchasing agency and the provider.

Another feature of this model is that it relies primarily on taxation to finance the health system. However, most middle income countries do not have a sufficiently large tax base to be able to finance a full basic package of health services from government budget alone. For this reason, it might be important to maintain the additional revenues from the GHI scheme.

Single payer system

Under this approach, the MOH will continue to function as the primary purchasing agent, possibly with two regional arms (one each for the West Bank and Gaza Strip) financed primarily through taxation and supplemented by health insurance premiums. However, the expansion of services will be achieved through contracting of services to private providers (e.g. non-profit organizations) rather than through direct expansion of the public delivery system. The major difference between this and the following social insurance model lies in the revenue source and governance structure of the purchasing agent. In a single payer system the purchasing agent remains a government agency which derives most of its revenues from taxation rather than from insurance premiums.

Social insurance model

This will involve the establishment of a separate social insurance agency, or a group of insurance agencies operating under a public mandate. A major portion of its revenues will be derived through insurance premiums, but the funds will also require subsidies through general revenues to equalize access for different subgroups within the population, e.g. the unemployed and low income households. This system has the advantage of clearly distinguishing the health insurance functions from the other government functions, and making the process of health financing more transparent to the public. However, it will also involve a major restructuring of the health financing system in order to establish an insurance agency or a sickness fund that is independent of the MOH. One potential drawback of this system is that in many middle income countries an independent social insurance agency or sickness funds have shown a tendency to develop its own, separate health delivery system paralleling the system financed directly by the MOH. It could lead to further fragmentation of the financing and delivery system, and to duplication and wastage of resources as well as inequities in access to services.

Table A 10.21, presents a schematic profile of the three types of health financing systems in which universal coverage has been achieved. There is no single "correct" path towards universal coverage: policy makers will need to weigh out the potential drawbacks and advantages of each approach and select the approach that is in keeping with the social and political values as well as economic capacities of the country.

Table A 10.21: Different Models of Health Financing and Management Systems

	Single Payer System	Integrated Health System	Social Insurance System
Examples	Canada - financed mainly by taxation with mainly private providers	UK / Scandinavian countries, Portugal - financed mainly by taxation with mainly public providers	Germany, France, Belgium - financed mainly by social insurance with mixed public and private providers Netherlands - financed by a mixture of social and private insurance with mainly private providers
Type of Public Purchasing Agency	Provincial, regional or local health authority	Ministry of Health, regional/local health authorities, municipalities	Sickness fund, social security agency
Main Source of Revenue	General tax revenues	General tax revenues	Payroll tax, employer and employee contributions
Typical Hospital Payment Systems	Contracts and other forms of provider payment system with autonomous providers	Direct administrative control with salaried personnel and budget transfers; increasingly, this system is being replaced by contracts with semi-autonomous public providers	Contracts, and other forms of prospective payment systems with autonomous providers (private and public)
Typical Physician Payment Systems	Fee-for-service with referrals required for specialist services	Salaried physicians; general practitioners, fundholding, fee-for-service with referrals required for specialist services	Fee-for-service, sometimes with balanced billing
Private Insurance	Mainly supplementary to public financing	Mainly supplementary to public financing	Mainly supplementary to social insurance; certain groups, e.g. the wealthy, are allowed to finance their health care services entirely from private insurance

Source: World Bank

ANNEX 1

List Of Persons Met

Ministry of Health
H.E. Dr. Riyad Zanoun, Minister
Dr. Munzer Sharif, Deputy Minister

West Bank
Dr. Fahed M. Es-Sayed, Director General, West Bank
Dr. Deib F. Ahmad, Director General, Health Insurance
Dr. Nabeel Idrees, Director, Health Insurance
Dr. Faisal Abdal-Latif, HRD Director
Mr. Mohamed Alyan, Director, Finance and Administration
Mr. Fouad Ghabbani, Director, Accounts Department
Mr. Samir Jabr, Finance Officer

Dr. Anan W.Masri, Director Watani Hospital
Dr. Omar Nasir, Assistant Director, Hospital Division
Mr. Walid Obeidallah, Assistant Director, Pharmaceutical Division

Gaza Strip
Dr. Yehia Abed, Director General, Research, Planning and Development
Dr. Mohammad Abu Hashish, Director General, Health Insurance
Dr. Faisal Abu Shahla, Director General, Hospital Directorate
Mr. Nasr Mohammad Nasr, Director, Financing
Mr. Abdul Fatah Al-Afifi, Project Coordinating Unit (PCU), Finance
Mr. Mithgal Fathi Abu-Ramadan, Assistant Accounting Manager, PCU

Ministry of Finance
Dr. Abu Husama Sa'id, Director General, Budget

Palestinian Central Bureau of Statistics
Dr. Hasan Abu-Libdeh, President

Private/NGO sector
Arabcare Medical
Dr. Rafiq Husseini, General Manager, Arabcare Medical Services

Patient Friendship Benevolent Society Gaza City
Dr. Hilmi Hammad, Director

Palestine Red Crescent Society - Khan Younis
Dr. Najjat, President, Khan Younis Branch

Trust International
Ms. Ranna Shunnar

Union of Palestinian Medical Relief Committee
Dr. Mustafa Barghouthi, President

Private Practitioner
Dr. Nafiz R. Abu-Shaban, Plastic Surgeon

UNRWA
West Bank
Dr. Arafat S. Hidmi, Chief, Field Health Programme
Ms. Randa Rantissi, Administrative Officer, Health Department

Gaza Strip
Dr. Ayyoub El-Alem, Chief, Field Health Programme, Gaza City
Ms. Inshirah El-Madhoun, Administrative Officer, Gaza City

UNICEF
Filippo Chiabrera, HSMU/ Project Manager

WHO
Dr. Paolo Piva, Resident Coordinator

American Jewish Joint Distribution Committee
Ms. Tamara Barnea, Director Special Programs in the Middle East
Dr. Bruce Rosen, Health Research Program

ANNEX 2

References

1. Barghouthi, M. and Lennock, J., "Health in Palestine: Potential and Challenges", MAS Discussion Papers, Palestine Economic Policy Research Institute (MAS), March 1997.

2. Chernichovsky, D., and Chinitz, D., "The Political Economy of Health System Reform in Israel," *Health Economics*, Vol. 4: 127-141, 1995.

3. Ismail, N.A., Alami, M. and Hammad, A., *Palestinian Universal Health Insurance: Questions and Answers*, Planning and Research Center, Jerusalem, August, 1994.

4. Palestinian Central Bureau of Statistics, *Bulletin of Consumer Prices: Average Prices for November - December, 1996*, Ramallah, West Bank, January 1997.

5. *Demographic Survey in the West Bank and Gaza*, Ramallah, West Bank, March 1996.

6. *Survey of Wages and Work Hours - 1994: Main Findings*, Ramallah, West Bank, December 1995.

7. United Nations Relief and Works Agency for Palestine Refugees in the Near East, Annual Report of the Department of Health, 1994 and 1995.

8. The World Bank, *Developing the Occupied Territories, An Investment in Peace, Human Resources and Social Policy*, Vol. 6, Washington, D.C., 1993.

9. Zavadjil, M., Calika, N., Kanaan, O., and Chua, D., "Recent Economic Developments: Prospects, and Progress in Institution Building in the West Bank and Gaza", International Monetary Fund, Middle East Department, Washington, D.C., 1997.

10. Palestinian Authority Ministry of Health, *The Status of Health in the Palestine. Annual Report 1996*. Prepared by Health Research & Planning Directorate, Statistics and Information Department. June 1997.

The Working Paper also drew upon numerous unpublished data and reports provided by the Ministry of Health, the Palestinian Central Bureau for Statistics, UNRWA, WHO and the World Bank.

ANNEX 3

Annex Table 3.1: West Bank and Gaza: National Health Expenditure, by Source of Revenues

	1991	1995	1996	1997 (estimation)
Government Health Insurance	42	24	22	27
General Revenues	0	45	67	61
UNRWA	13	29	23	30
Donor Contributions	77	25	44	31
NGOs (estimated for 1996-97)	0	37	20	10
Private Household and Corporations	91	108	102	105
Total	223	268	278	264
Percent Growth Rate (nominal)			3.7	-5
Population, Thousands	1,800	2,151	2,280	2,372
Per capita Health Expenditure, US$	124	125	122	111
Percentage Distribution				
Government Health Insurance	19	9	8	10
General Revenues	0	17	24	23
UNRWA	6	11	8	11
Donor Contributions	35	9	16	12
NGOs	0	14	7	4
Private	41	40	37	40
Total	100	100	100	100
Total Revenues (IMF figures)		424.9	670.1	814.2
Israeli Health Fees (IMF figures)		10.1	5.4	7.1
Israeli Health Fees(MOH figures)		8.2	8.2	
		69.2	88.6	87.5
General Revenues		45.1	67.1	60.6
Health Insurance		24.1	21.5	26.9
		16.3%	13.2%	10.8%

Source: Ministry of Health, United Nations Relief and Work Agency for Palestine Refugees in the Near East,International Monetary Fund, PCBS, World Bank Staff Calculations.

ANNEX 4

Annex Table 4.1: West Bank and Gaza: Ministry of Health Expenditures

		1993	1994	1995	1996	1997 /1
US$ (thousand)						
Salaries		19,514	Not Available	37,567	42,833	40,031
Overseas Treatment		11,702	Not Available	14,114	15,707	15,000
Drug and Disposable		21,498	Not Available	16,656	28,178	31,533
Food		0	Not Available	0	1,945	2,250
Operating Expenditures		9,262	Not Available	9,071	9,927	8,123
Total Expenditure		61,976	Not Available	77,408	98,590	96,937
Percent distribution						
Salaries		31.5	Not Available	48.5	43.4	41.3
Overseas Treatment		18.9	Not Available	18.2	15.9	15.5
Drug & Disposable		34.7	Not Available	21.5	28.6	32.5
Food		0.0	Not Available	0.0	2.0	2.3
Operating Expenditures		14.9	Not Available	11.7	10.1	8.4
Total		100.0		100.0	100.0	100.0

1. Ministry of Health projection
Source: Ministry of Health, 1997.

ANNEX 5

Government Health Insurance

Premium levels. Health insurance premium levels for different categories of beneficiaries are summarized in
Annex Table 5.1, below. Premium levels are set at approximately 5 percent of basic wage rate, with a minimum of NIS 40 and a maximum cap of NIS 75 per month per household. Recent attempts to increase the cap on the government employees to NIS 85 per month was rejected by the Cabinet, but the ceiling on voluntary contributions have been raised to NIS 85 per month in some cases.
Annex Table 5.2 shows the additional premiums charged for dependents of the head of the household.

Annex Table 5.1: Government Health Insurance Scheme: Premiums for Different Categories of Beneficiaries

Beneficiary Category	Basic Monthly Premium
Compulsory - Government Employees	5 percent of basic salary, with lower limit of NIS 40 and upper limit of NIS 75.
Voluntary - Individual Households	NIS 75 per household. NIS 50 for single individual.
Group Contracts Formally Employed (i.e. those with contracts and on a regular payroll)	5 percent of basic salary, deducted directly from the payroll - disclosure of payroll required; NIS 40 - 85.
Self-employed Groups - Groups Over 100	NIS 60 in Gaza Strip.
- Groups Under 100	NIS 65 in Gaza Strip.
Social Welfare Cases and Unemployed Workers	NIS 40. Social welfare cases must be validated by the social worker, and if approved, the premium for the eligible beneficiaries are, in principle, paid by Ministry of Social Welfare to the MOH.
Workers in Israel	NIS 93 - Workers who are employed more than 15 days in a month have premiums deducted directly from payroll by the Israeli Government, and collected fees are transferred to PA.
Students over 18 years of Age	NIS 20 in Gaza Strip.

Source: Health Insurance Department, Ministry of Health, Gaza City and Ramallah, 1997.

Annex Table 5.2: Government Health Insurance Scheme: Additional Premium Charged for Dependents

Category of Beneficiaries	Additional Monthly Premium
Spouses and Children under 18	Included in the basic premium.
Parents of the Head of Household	NIS 15 additional for parents over 60 years of age.
Additional First-degree Dependents	NIS 35 for more than two persons including parents.

Source: Health Insurance Department, Ministry of Health, Gaza City, 1997.

Copayment rates. All users of government health services are required to make copayments for drugs and diagnostic tests (see Table 5.3). Copayments in the amount of NIS 1 was recently introduced for the treatment of children under the age of three, where formerly they had been free of charge (see the Pharmaceutical Sector Report). Copayments are not required for emergency cases and for cases referred from government primary health care centers to government hospitals. At present there are no financial penalties for those who choose to skip the primary care physicians and coming straight to the hospital emergency unit for a non-emergency visit.

There is anecdotal evidence of the indigent households who face difficulties in making the copayments for the use of government health services. Whether these copayment levels actually result in denial of care for the social welfare cases will require further study.

Annex Table 5.3: MOH Facilities - Copayment Rates

Service Category	Copayment Rates
All Patients:	
Drugs	NIS 3 per prescription
- Children under 3 Years	NIS 1 per prescription
Laboratory Diagnostics	NIS 1 per request
Referral from:	
- Private Practitioner	NIS 20
Insured Patients:	
Laboratory Diagnostics and X-Ray	NIS 1 per request
Referral From:	
- Government Primary Care Provider	Free
Emergency Care at Government Hospitals	Free
Overseas Referrals	Variable contributions from patients - voluntary insurance holders are asked to contribute about a quarter of the total cost of referral.
Hospitalization and Associated Costs	Free

Source: Health Insurance Department, Ministry of Health, Gaza City, 1997.

Annex Table 5.3: Government Services Available for Insured and Uninsured Population

Population Group	Type of Services Covered
Personal Care for All Population (Insured and Uninsured)	<ul><li>Immunization</li><li>Antenatal and postnatal care</li><li>Preventive and curative care for all children under the age of three</li><li>Basic ambulatory (preventive) services</li><li>Hospital psychiatric services and community mental health program</li></ul>
Public Health Programs	<ul><li>School health services: preventive and basic treatment during school hours</li><li>Public environmental health program</li></ul>
Benefits for Insured Population	<ul><li>Primary curative care</li><li>Secondary care: hospitalization, including rehabilitation</li><li>Tertiary care, including overseas treatment or referrals to local private providers</li></ul>

Source: Ministry of Health, 1997.

Benefit. Table 5.4 summarizes the types of services covered by the government. Government provides public health programs and preventive health care free of charge for all citizens. Children under three have free access[63] to both preventive and curative care, but only insured patients above the age of three have free access to curative care. As noted earlier, the MOH's role as a third-party payer is limited to overseas referral cases and a few specialized cases approved for local referrals. There is, as yet, little complementarity between government and private or NGO services: MOH does not reimburse GHI patients for visits to private doctors and admissions to private or NGO hospitals (except for the special cases approved by the MOH's Medical Referral Committee). Hence, access to the benefits listed in Table 4 are effectively limited by the services available through the government health facilities.

Conversely, uninsured patients must pay the full cost of services for admissions to government hospitals. Per diem costs at government hospitals range from about NIS 200 per day

---

[63] Government health services are not entirely "free", since all patients, including those who are insured, are required to make copayments for drugs and diagnostic tests.

for pediatric care to over NIS 600 per day for intensive care. These fees represent a substantial cost to households, whose average monthly expenditure in 1996 was around NIS 2,610.[64]

Annex Table 5.5: West Bank and Gaza Government Health Insurance System

	Actual				Estimates
	1993	1994	1995	1996	Q1 1997
Health Insurance: Number of Insured Families					
West Bank and Gaza					
Type of Health Insurance Participants					
Voluntary - Individual	16,579	19,221	24,813	30,284	33,598
Group Contracts	0	6,074	19,157	24,069	40,439
Compulsory	22,321	27,916	31,815	36,980	41,582
Workers in Israel	31,120	20,648	20,713	25,008	26,565
Social Welfare Group	21,539	23,568	27,190	31,666	35,174
Total	91,559	97,427	123,688	148,007	177,358
West Bank					
Type of Health Insurance Participants					
Voluntary - Individual	6,206	6,191	9,275	13,263	14,462
Group Contracts		2,559	9,931	11,991	24,034
Compulsory (government employees)	15,105	16,633	19,331	22,781	25,742
Workers in Israel	13,961	10,949	8,122	10,261	10,483
Social Welfare Group	11,539	12,056	12,181	15,924	17,524
Total	46,811	48,388	58,840	74,220	92,245
Gaza Strip					
Type of Health Insurance Participants					
Voluntary - Individual	10,373	13,030	15,538	17,021	19,136
Group Contracts		3,515	9,226	12,078	16,405
Compulsory (government employees)	7,216	11,283	12,484	14,199	15,840
Workers in Israel	17,159	9,699	12,591	14,747	16,082
Social Welfare Group	10,000	11,512	15,009	15,742	17,650
Total	44,748	49,039	64,848	73,787	85,113
Health Insurance: Number of Insured Individuals					
West Bank and Gaza					
Type of Health Insurance Participants					
Voluntary - Individual and Group	0	0	215,200	264,958	359,863
Compulsory (government employees)	0	0	151,906	176,349	199,486
Workers in Israel			102,022	122,859	147,195
Social Welfare Group			97,514	112,351	123,058
Total			566,643	676,517	829,603
Population Insured	0 %	0 %	26.3 %	29,7 %	35 %
West Bank					
Type of Health Insurance Participants					
Voluntary - Individual and Group			86,427	113,643	175,050
Compulsory			86,990	102,515	117,118
Workers in Israel			36,549	46,175	63,569
Social Welfare Group			38,979	50,957	54,223
Total	0	0	248,945	313,289	409,960
Population Insured	0%	0%	20%	24%	30%

---

[64] Palestinian Expenditure and Consumption Survey, October 1995 - September 1996, Palestinian Central Statistical Bureau, 1996.

Annex Table 5.5 continued

Gaza Strip					
Type of Health Insurance Participants					
Voluntary - Individual and Group			128,773	151,315	184,813
Compulsory			64,917	73,835	82,368
Workers in Israel			65,473	76,684	83,626
Social Welfare Group			58,535	61,394	68,835
Total	0	0	317,698	363,22	419,643
Population Insured	0 %	0 %	35 %	38 %[8]	44 %
Insurance revenues (NIS, thousands)					
West Bank and Gaza					
Type of Health Insurance Participants					
Voluntary -Individual		13,848	12,666		
Contract (group)			4,684	11,196	
Compulsory			29,151	23,718	
Workers in Israel			24,665	24,086	
Social Welfare Group			0	0	
Copayments (stamps)			8,085	9,757	
Total			80,433	81,422	
West Bank					
Type of Health Insurance Participants					
Voluntary - Individual			7,972	8,349	
Voluntary - Group			4,477	8,174	
Compulsory			20,042	12,954	
Workers in Israel			9,744	11,969	
Social Welfare Group			0	0	
Copayment (stamps)			4,012	4,585	
Total			46,247	46,031	
Gaza Strip					
Type of Health Insurance Participants					
Voluntary - Individual	6,194	5,226	5,876	4,317	
Contract (group)		386	207	3,022	
Compulsory (Government employees)	6,864	5,757	9,109	10,764	
Workers in Israel	16,581	14,753	14,921	12,117	
Social Welfare Group	0	0	0	0	
Copayment (stamps)		2,506	4,073	5,172	
Total	29,639	28,628	34,186	35,391	
Insurance revenues (US$ thousands)					
West Bank and Gaza					
Type of Health Insurance Participants					
Voluntary			6,178	7,231	
Compulsory (government employees)			4.77	4.77	
Workers in Israel			8,222	7,299	
Social Welfare Group			0	0	
Total			24,117	21,716	
West Bank					
Type of Health Insurance Participants					
Voluntary			4,150	5,007	
Compulsory (government employees)			6,681	3,925	
Workers in Israel			3,248	3,627	
Social Welfare Group			0	0	
Total			14,079	12,559	

Annex Table 5.5 continued

Gaza Strip
Type of Health Insurance Participants

Voluntary	2,028	2,224
Compulsory (government employees)	3,036	3,261
Workers in Israel	4,974	3,672
Social Welfare Group	0	0
Total	10,038	9,157

Contributions per Family per Year, by Different Types (US$)
West Bank and Gaza
Type of Health Insurance Participants

Voluntary	141	133
Compulsory (government employees)	305	194
Workers in Israel	397	292
Social Welfare group	0	0

West Bank
Type of Health Insurance Participants

Voluntary	216	198
Compulsory (government employees)	346	172
Workers in Israel	400	353
Social Welfare Group	0	0

Gaza Strip
Type of Health Insurance Participants

Voluntary	82	76
Compulsory (government employees)	243	230
Workers in Israel	395	249
Social Welfare Group	0	0

Average Number of Beneficiaries per Family Unit
West Bank and Gaza
Type of Health Insurance Participants

Voluntary	4.89	4.87
Compulsory (government employees)	4.77	4.77
Workers in Israel	4.93	4.91
Social Welfare Group	3.59	3.55

West Bank
Type of Health Insurance Participants

Voluntary	4.50	4.50
Compulsory (government employees)	4.50	4.50
Workers in Israel	4.50	4.50
Social Welfare Group	3.20	3.20

Gaza Strip
Type of Health Insurance Participants

Voluntary	5.20	5.20
Compulsory (government employees)	5.20	5.20
Workers in Israel	5.20	5.20
Social Welfare Group	3.90	3.90

Source: Ministry of Health, Health Insurance Department, 1997.

ANNEX 6

Annex Table 6.1: West Bank and Gaza Health Facilities, 1997
Summary of Health Facilities and Services

Facility Types, by Sector	Number of Existing Facilities			Proposed New Facilities			Investment (US$ millions)			Acute Care Geds		Chronic Care Beds
	Hospitals	Clinics	Other	Hospitals	Clinics	Other	New	Rehabilitation	Equipment	Existing	Proposed	
Ministry of Health												
West Bank												
Hospitals												
Secondary/Tertiary	8			2			130.0	4.6	3.9	708	740	
Psychiatric Hospital	1							3.2				320
Clinics												
PHC Centers		178										
MCH Clinics		9										
Village Health Rooms			74									
Ambulance Services							5.0					
Nursing School						1	1.5					
Central Stores						1	2.5					
Central Maintenance Workshop						1	0.25					
Gaza Strip												
Hospitals												
Secondary/Tertiary	5			3			56.4	1.0	6.1	751	217	
Psychiatric	1											34
Primary Health Care Centers		31			5							
West Bank and Gaza												
PHC Equipment									11.4			
Hospital Equipment									33.2			
Public Health Lab (Ramallah and Gaza)						1	2.8					
Subtotals, Ministry of Health				5	5	4	195.6	8.8	54.6	1,459	957	354
UNRWA												
West Bank												
Hospital												
Qalqilya	1						2.0			43	20	0
Subcontract	4									*125*		
Reimbursement	N/A											
Clinics												
Health Centers		22										
Health Points		12										
Dental Clinics		17										
Special Care (noncom)		34										
Laboratories			19									

Annex Table 6.1 continued

Gaza Strip												
Hospital												
European Gaza				1			55.0				200	
Subcontract (al-Ahli)	1									*50*		
Reimbursement												
Clinics												
Health Centers		11										
Health Points		1										
MCH Centers		6										
Dental Clinics		12										
Special Care (noncom)		11										
Laboratories			11									
Subtotals, UNRWA							57.0	.		43	220	0
Nongovernmental Organizations Sector												
E. Jerusalem												
Hospitals												
Tertiary (Maqassad)	1									264		
Secondary	4									296		
West Bank												
Acute Care Hospitals	7									352		
Maternity Clinics	9									115		
Rehabilitation Clinics	2											72
Clinics		176										
Gaza Strip												
Acute Care Hospitals	2			1			15			116	120	
Clinics		31			5							
Subtotals, Nongovernmental Organizations				1	5		15			583	120	72
Private Sector							40.0					
West Bank												
Hospitals				2							168	
Maternity	7									79		
Clinics		164								30	20	
Diagnostic Unit				1	2							
Specialized Centers				1	1	1						
Gaza Strip												
Hospitals												
Maternity	2									37		
Clinics												
Diagnostic Unit												
Subtotals, Private Sector				2	3	1	40			146	188	0
Total, All Sectors (Excluding East Jerusalem)							250.6	8.8	54.6	2,231	1,485	426
Total, All Sectors (Including East Jerusalem)										2,791		

ANNEX 7

Annex Table 7.1: West Bank and Gaza Strip: Inpatient Discharge Rates

	Actual		Percent
	1995	**1996**	**Change**
Total Population Size (in thousands)	2,151	2,280	6
Total Number of Patient Discharge	78,009	199,271	12
Government Hospital Patients	151,740/[1]	156,936	3
NGO West Bank Patients	25,261	32,092	27
NGO Gaza Patients (al-Ahli-Arabi)		6,310	
UNRWA Qalqilya	1,008	3,933	290
Inpatient Discharge Rates as Percent of Population/[2]	8.3	8.7	6
Number of Overseas Cases	4,417	6,476	47
Overseas Cases as Percent of Total Inpatient Cases	2.5	3.2	31
Overseas Cases as Percent of Total Population	0.2	0.3	38
Total Inpatient Discharge Rates	8.5	9.0	6

1. This figure includes the discharges from Ahli-Arabi (NGO) Hospital in Gaza
2. This figure to some extend under-reports the total discharge rates, since patients admitted to small NGO clinics and some private hospitals are not included.
Source: Compiled from data provided by the MOH, Nablus and Gaza City, 1997.

Annex Table 7.2: West Bank and Gaza Strip: Hospital Utilization Data - Summary

	1994	1995	1996	Percent change 1995~96
Ministry of Health Hospitals				
West Bank (excludes psychiatric hospital				
Total Beds		706	728	3.1
Total Discharges		78,302	82,694	5.6
Average Length of Stay (days)		2.6	2.8	7.5
Bed Occupancy Rate (percent)		79	84	6.5
OPD		408,489	530,431	29.9
Operations (major and minor)		Not Available	21,461	Not Available
Gaza Strip				
Total Beds	840	840	929	0.0
Total Discharges	65,591	73,438	79,981	8.9
Average Length of Stay (days)	3.3	3.2	3.4	6.2
Bed Occupancy Rate (percent)	71	76	81	6.6
OPD	..	286,561	318,826	11.3
Emergency	86,731	117,138	142,517	21.7
Major Operations	10,364	126,24	12,674	0.4
NGO Sector				
West Bank				
General Hospitals				
Total Beds		331	332	0.3
Total Discharges		22,906	25,185	9.9
Average Length of Stay (days)		3.1	3.1	1.1
Bed Occupancy Rate (percent)		59	64	8.1
OPD		76,493	76,127	-0.5
Operations		6,088	7,360	20.9
NGO Maternity Hospitals				
Total Beds		112	115	2.7
Total Discharges		7,670	7,853	2.4
Average Length of Stay (days)		1.4	1.2	-13.3
Bed Occupancy Rate (percent)		26	24	-6.2
OPD		8,673	1,905	-78.0
Operations		1,688	569	-66.3
Gaza Strip				
Total Beds		38	218	
UNRWA Qalqilya Hospital				
Total Beds		38	38	0.0
Total Discharges		3,363	3,933	16.9
Average Length of Stay (days)		2.8	4.0	43.1

Annex Table 7.2 continued

Bed Occupancy Rate (percent)		69	114	65.1
OPD		29,833	36,043	20.8
Operations		914	1,446	58.2
Summary Table for 1996				
Acute Care Hospitals		**Beds**	**Discharges**	**Percent Bed**
MOH Hospitals		1,479	155,763	71
NGO Hospitals/Clinics		563	38,936	27
UNRWA		38	3,933	2
East Jerusalem NGO Hospitals		560		
Total without East Jerusalem		2,080	198,632	
Total with East Jerusalem		2,640		

Source: Ministry of Health, World Bank Staff Calculations.

ANNEX 8

West Bank And Gaza: Hospital Cost Analysis

The unit costs of government hospitals in West Bank were estimated on the basis of the 1996 detailed recurrent expenditure and utilization data provided by the MOH, Nablus. Capital depreciation costs are not included in these estimates.

In the absence of detailed cost accounting data, the relative values were assigned to distribute the costs by different categories of hospital services as indicated in Table 8.1. In other words, it is assumed that the average cost of one inpatient day is about three times the average cost of outpatient care, and so forth.

Annex Table 8.1: Allocation of Relative Values to Various Hospital Service Activities

Service Category	Relative Value
Inpatient Day	3.0
Outpatient Visit (treatment without hospitalization admission)	1.0
Day-Care Patient (day-beds)	2.0
Emergency Visit	0.5

Source: World Bank Staff Estimates.

Using this allocation rule, the unit cost of each category of service was calculated for each of the government hospitals in West Bank. The results are summarized in Table 8.2, and the details are presented in Table 8.3. The MOH estimated that the average annual running cost of government hospitals to be around $26,836, which is in close conformity with the figure obtained below[65].

Annex Table 8.2: Average Unit Cost Estimates for Government Hospitals in West Bank

	NIS	US$
Cost per Patient Day	149	47
Cost per Outpatient Visit	50	16
Cost per Emergency	25	8
Cost per Bed per Year	90,241	28,378

Source: World Bank Staff Estimates.

A comparison of the relative costs of government hospitals shown in Table 8.3 reveals some of the differences in the relative efficiency of each of these hospitals. Tulkarem and Jericho hospitals have the lowest cost per bed, reflecting the limited number and level of specialized care offered at these facilities. However, the cost of inpatient day at Jericho hospital is as high as the cost of inpatient day at Beit Jalla hospital - a more comprehensive hospital - due to the low bed occupancy rate at Jericho hospital which raises the unit cost of service. These unit cost measures presented here in are very crude and require further refinements and verifications by more detailed financial analysis of each hospitals including cost accounting and utilization studies. Nonetheless, they begin to reveal some of the underlying inefficiencies and differences in the productivity of the individual hospitals.

---

[65] Cited in Barghouthi and Lennock, 1997, p. 37.

Annex Table 8.3: West Bank and Gaza Strip - Government and UNRWA Hospital Costs, 1996

Facility	Location	Number of Beds	Bed Occupancy Rate (percent)	Total Revenues/1 (NIS)	Revenues as Percent Expenditure	Total Expenditure (NIS)	Staff Costs (NIS)	Staff Cost as Percent of Expenditure	Unit Costs (NIS) Cost per Patient-Day	Cost per Day-Care	Cost per Emergency	Cost per Visit	Cost per Bed	Cost/Bed (US$)
West Bank Government Hospital Sector														
Acute Care Hospitals														
Beit Jala Government Hospital	Bethlehem	70	82	712,023	9	7,542,823	2,905,568	39	152	N/A.	25	51	107,755	$33,885
Hebron Government Hospital	Hebron	103	102	1,375,818	14	10,071,233	4,385,999	44	119	79	20	40	97,779	$30,748
Jenin Government Hospital	Jenin	55	118	1,194,644	22	5,532,293	2,702,826	49	131	N/A.	22	44	100,587	$31,631
Jericho Government Hospital	Jericho	50	49	385,273	10	3,769,688	1,678,607	45	158	N/A.	26	53	75,394	$23,709
Al-Watani Hospital	Nablus	86	69	290,052	4	8,099,386	3,082,026	38	175	117	29	58	94,179	$29,616
Rafidia Hospital	Nablus	138	83	2,000,563	19	10,618,059	4,906,911	46	148	N/A.	25	49	76,942	$24,196
Ramallah Government Hospital	Ramallah	142	83	1,234,650	8	15,108,166	5,533,195	37	169	113	28	56	106,396	$33,458
Tulkarem Government Hospital	Tulkarem	84	80	757,907	15	4,954,093	2,723,024	55	128	N/A.	21	43	58,977	$18,546
Total / *Weighted Average*		**728**	**84**	**7,950,930**	**12**	**65,695,741**	**27,918,156**	**42**	**149**		**25**	**50**	**90,241**	**$28,378**
Psychiatric Care														
Kamal Psychiatric Hospital	Bethlehem	320	109	15,969	0.4	4,114,896	2,549,733	62	32			8	12,859	$4,044
UNRWA Qalqilya Hospital														
UNRWA	Qalqilya	38	113			3,219,263	2,451,627	76	130			32	84,717	$26,641

Sources: For government hospitals, 1996 hospital expenditure data were provided by the MOH, Nablus, West Bank. For UNRWA Qalqilya hospital, data were provided by UNRWA West Bank Field Office, E. Jerusalem.

ANNEX 9

Annex Table 9.1: West Bank and Gaza: Public Investment Plan for the Health Sector, 1997-2002 (US$ millions, constant 1997 price)

	1997	1998	1999	2000	2001	2002
Hospitals (includes psychiatric hospital)	35.1	35.1	35.1	35.1	35.1	35.1
Building	28.1	28.1	28.1	28.1	28.1	28.1
Upgrading, Rehabilitation	1.5	1.5	1.5	1.5	1.5	1.5
Equipment	5.5	5.5	5.5	5.5	5.5	5.5
Primary Health Care Centers	11.1	8.5	8.5	6.9	4.2	4.0
Building	9.2	6.6	6.1	4.5	2.3	2.1
Rehabilitation/ Renovation	0	0	0.5	0.5	0	0
Equipment	1.9	1.9	1.9	1.9	1.9	1.9
Other Investments:/1	2.0	2.0	2.0	2.0	2.0	2.0
Public Health Laboratory						
Ambulance Services						
Nursing School (3000 sqm)						
Central Stores (6000 sqm)						
Central Maintenance Workshop (500 sqm.)						
Total	48.2	45.6	45.6	44.0	41.3	41.1

Source: Ministry of Health

Annex Table 9.2: West Bank and Gaza: Recurrent Cost Estimates for the New Facilities, 1997-2002 (US$ millions, constant 1997 price)

	1997	1998	1999	2000	2001	2002
Projection I (higher projection)						
Hospital Sector at 25 Percent of Investment	8.4	16.8	25.2	33.6	42.0	50.4
Recurrent Cost of EU Hospital /1	0.0	5.3	10.5	10.5	10.5	10.5
Primary Health Care Sector at 40 Percent Investment	4.4	7.8	11.2	14.0	15.6	17.2
Subtotal	12.8	29.9	47.0	58.1	68.2	78.2
Projection II (lower projection)						
Hospital Sector at 20 Percent of Investment	6.7	13.4	20.2	26.9	33.6	40.3
Recurrent Cost of EU Hospital / 1	0.0	4.2	8.4	8.4	8.4	8.4
Primary Health Care Sector at 30 Percent Investment	3.3	5.9	8.4	10.5	11.7	12.9
Subtotal	10.0	23.5	37.0	45.8	53.8	61.7
Projection III: Average of I and II						
Hospital Sector	7.6	15.1	22.7	30.3	37.8	45.4
Recurrent Cost of EU Hospital /1	0.0	4.7	9.5	9.5	9.5	9.5
Primary Health Care Sector	3.9	6.8	9.8	12.2	13.7	15.1
Subtotal	11.4	26.7	42.0	52.0	61.0	69.9

1. EU Hospital is treated separated since the investment cost in EU is not included in the above estimates for years 1997-2002. It is assumed that 100 beds will become operational in 1998 and the remaining 100 beds in 1999. Since the exact timing of investments are not known for this category, the estimated total was divided equally across the years, 1997-2002.
Source: Ministry of Health, World Bank Staff Estimates.

ANNEX 10

Annex Table 10.1: West Bank and Gaza: Projected Inpatient Bed Requirements 1997-2002 at Various Admission Rates, Bed Occupancy Rates and Length of Stay

	1997	1998	1999	2000	2001	2002	Average Annual Increment
Population (thousand)	2,372	2,467	2,565	2,668	2,775	2,886	86
Number of Expected Patients							
7 Percent Admission Rate	166,040	172,690	179,550	186,760	194,230	202,000	5,993
8 Percent Admission Rate	189,760	197,360	205,200	213,440	221,978	230,857	6,849
9 Percent Admission Rate	213,480	222,030	230,850	240,120	249,725	259,714	7,706
10 Percent Admission Rate	237,200	246,700	256,500	266,800	277,472	288,571	8,562
Patient Days							
ALOS of 3 Days							
7 Percent Admission Rate	498,120	518,070	538,650	560,280	582,691	605,999	17,980
8 Percent Admission Rate	569,280	592,080	615,600	640,320	665,933	692,570	20,548
9 Percent Admission Rate	640,440	666,090	692,550	720,360	749,174	779,141	23,117
10 Percent Admission Rate	711,600	740,100	769,500	800,400	832,416	865,713	25,685
ALOS of 4 Days							
8 Percent Admission Rate	759,040	789,440	820,800	853,760	887,910	923,427	27,398
9 Percent Admission Rate	853,920	888,120	923,400	960,480	998,899	1,038,855	30,823
10 Percent Admission Rate	948,800	986,800	1,026,000	1,067,200	1,109,888	1,154,284	34,247
ALOS of 5 Days							
8 Percent Admission Rate	948,800	986,800	1,026,000	1,067,200	1,109,888	1,154,284	34,247
9 Percent Admission Rate	1,067,400	1,110,150	1,154,250	1,200,600	1,248,624	1,298,569	38,528
10 Percent Admission Rate	1,186,000	1,233,500	1,282,500	1,334,000	1,387,360	1,442,854	42,809
Days per Bed Available per Year							
80 Percent Occupancy Rate	292	292	292	292	292	292	-
70 Percent Occupancy Rate	256	256	256	256	256	256	-
60 Percent Occupancy Rate	219	219	219	219	219	219	-
Hospital Bed Requirements							
Assuming 80 Percent Occupancy Rate							
ALOS of 3 Days							
7 Percent Admission Rate	1,706	1,774	1,845	1,919	1,996	2,075	62
8 Percent Admission Rate	1,950	2,028	2,108	2,193	2,281	2,372	70
9 Percent Admission Rate	2,193	2,281	2,372	2,467	2,566	2,668	79
10 Percent Admission Rate	2,437	2,535	2,635	2,741	2,851	2,965	88
ALOS of 4 Days							
8 Percent Admission Rate	2,599	2,704	2,811	2,924	3,041	3,162	94
9 Percent Admission Rate	2,924	3,042	3,162	3,289	3,421	3,558	106
10 Percent Admission Rate	3,249	3,379	3,514	3,655	3,801	3,953	117
ALOS of 5 Days							
8 Percent Admission Rate	3,249	3,379	3,514	3,655	3,801	3,953	117
9 Percent Admission Rate	3,655	3,802	3,953	4,112	4,276	4,447	132
10 Percent Admission Rate	4,062	4,224	4,392	4,568	4,751	4,941	147
Assuming 70 Percent occupancy rate							
ALOS of 3 Days							
7 Percent Admission Rate	1,950	2,028	2,108	2,193	2,281	2,372	70
8 Percent Admission Rate	2,228	2,317	2,409	2,506	2,606	2,711	80
9 Percent Admission Rate	2,507	2,607	2,711	2,819	2,932	3,049	90
10 Percent Admission Rate	2,785	2,897	3,012	3,133	3,258	3,388	101

Annex Table 10.1 continued

ALOS of 4 Days							
8 Percent Admission Rate	2,971	3,090	3,213	3,342	3,475	3,614	107
9 Percent Admission Rate	3,342	3,476	3,614	3,759	3,910	4,066	121
10 Percent Admission Rate	3,714	3,862	4,016	4,177	4,344	4,518	134
ALOS of 5 Days							
8 Percent Admission Rate	3,714	3,862	4,016	4,177	4,344	4,518	134
9 Percent Admission Rate	4,178	4,345	4,518	4,699	4,887	5,082	151
10 Percent Admission Rate	4,642	4,828	5,020	5,221	5,430	5,647	168
Beds per 1,000 Population							
Assuming 80 Percent occupancy rate							
ALOS of 3 Days							
7 Percent Admission Rate	0.7	0.7	0.7	0.7	0.7	0.7	-
8 Percent Admission Rate	0.8	0.8	0.8	0.8	0.8	0.8	-
9 Percent Admission Rate	0.9	0.9	0.9	0.9	0.9	0.9	-
10 Percent Admission Rate	1.0	1.0	1.0	1.0	1.0	1.0	-
ALOS of 4 Days							
8 Percent Admission Rate	1.1	1.1	1.1	1.1	1.1	1.1	-
9 Percent Admission Rate	1.2	1.2	1.2	1.2	1.2	1.2	-
10 Percent Admission Rate	1.4	1.4	1.4	1.4	1.4	1.4	-
ALOS of 5 Days							
8 Percent Admission Rate	1.4	1.4	1.4	1.4	1.4	1.4	-
9 Percent Admission Rate	1.5	1.5	1.5	1.5	1.5	1.5	-
10 Percent Admission Rate	1.7	1.7	1.7	1.7	1.7	1.7	-
Assuming 70 Percent occupancy rate							
ALOS of 3 Days							
8 Percent Admission Rate	0.9	0.9	0.9	0.9	0.9	0.9	-
9 Percent Admission Rate	1.1	1.1	1.1	1.1	1.1	1.1	-
10 Percent Admission Rate	1.2	1.2	1.2	1.2	1.2	1.2	-
ALOS of 4 Days							
8 Percent Admission Rate	1.3	1.3	1.3	1.3	1.3	1.3	-
9 Percent Admission Rate	1.4	1.4	1.4	1.4	1.4	1.4	-
10 Percent Admission Rate	1.6	1.6	1.6	1.6	1.6	1.6	-
ALOS of 5 Days							
8 Percent Admission Rate	1.6	1.6	1.6	1.6	1.6	1.6	-
9 Percent Admission Rate	1.8	1.8	1.8	1.8	1.8	1.8	-
10 Percent Admission Rate	2.0	2.0	2.0	2.0	2.0	2.0	-

Source: Ministry of Health, World Bank Staff Estimates.

ANNEX 11

Annex Table 11.1: West Bank and Gaza: Number of Outpatient Visits, 1996

	Population	Outpatient		Visits per Person (per Year)	
		Number of Visits	Percent	Refugee Population	Total Population
Total Population (thousand), 1997	2,280,000				
West Bank	1,370,000				
Gaza Strip	1,002,000				
Refugee Population	1,299,732				
West Bank	553,868				
Gaza Strip	745,864				
Total Outpatient Visits		8,808,123	100		3.9
Total Visits to Ministry of Health		3,499,577	40		1.53
West Bank Hospitals		530,431	6		
West Bank Public Health Services		1,507,732	17		
Gaza Strip Hospitals		230,609	3		
Gaza Strip Public Health Services		1,230,805	14		.
Total Visits to NGO Hospitals		103,055	1		0.05
Total Visits to Private Practice		2,736,000	31		1.20/a
Total Visits to UNRWA/b		2,469,491	28	1.9/b	

a. Based on the household expenditure figure of about $9 per individual, compared with each physician consultations which cost around $15, based on the recommended fee schedule from the Palestinian Medical Association. From these figures we estimate $9/$15 = 0.6 contacts per individual, or 1.2 visits per person if we assume on average about 1 repeat visit (free of charge) for each physician contact.

b. The approximate visits per person for UNRWA services were calculated from following 1995 figures:

UNRWA Outpatient Visits	
West Bank	
Number of Outpatient Visits	811,120
Refugee Population	524,000
Visits per Person	1.5
Gaza Strip	
Number of Outpatient Visits	1,525,675
Refugee Population	701,000
Visits per Person	2.2
Total: West Bank and Gaza	
Number of Outpatient Visits	2,336,795
Refugee Population	1,225,000
Visits per Person	1.9

Source: UNRWA 1995 Annual Report of the Department of Health.

ANNEX 12

Annex Table 12.1: West Bank and Gaza: Monthly Household Expenditures October 1995-September 1996 (JD = 4.41 NIS - US$ = 3.15 NIS)

	Average Size of Households	Monthly Household Expenditures						Medical Care as Percent of Total Expenditure	Per Capita Monthly Expenditure (US$)		Annual per Capita Household Expenditure (US$)	
		Medical Care /a			Total Household Expenditure				Medical	Total	Medical	Total
		JD	NIS	US$	JD	NIS	US$					
West Bank and Gaza	6.9	20.6	91	29	592	2,610	828	3.5	4.2	120	50	1,440
Location												
Camp	7.4	13.51	60	19	488	2,150	682	2.8	2.6	92	31	1,106
Village	7	23.26	102	33	590	2,600	825	3.9	4.6	118	56	1,414
City	6.8	20.16	89	28	635	2,796	887	3.2	4.1	130	50	1,565
Governorates												
Gaza Strip	8.0	13.86	61	19	503	2,215	703	2.8	2.4	88	29	1,054
West Bank	6.5	23.32	103	33	629	2,770	879	3.7	5.0	135	60	1,622
South	7.2	27.22	120	38	582	2,565	814	4.7	5.3	113	63	1,356
Middle	6.3	22.57	99	32	760	3,349	1,062	3.0	5.0	169	60	2,024
North	6.2	21.22	93	30	573	2,525	801	3.7	4.8	129	57	1,550
Bethlehem		28.33	125	40	670	2,953	937	4.2	Not Available	Not Available	Not Available	Not Available
Hebron		26.81	118	37	550	2,424	769	4.9	Not Available	Not Available	Not Available	Not Available
Jerusalem		20.98	92	29	836	3,684	1,169	2.5	Not Available	Not Available	Not Available	Not Available
Ramallah/ Jericho		23.64	104	33	709	3,123	991	3.3	Not Available	Not Available	Not Available	Not Available
Tulkarem/ Qalqilya		21.98	97	31	549	2,419	767	4.0	Not Available	Not Available	Not Available	Not Available
Nablus		22.04	97	31	592	2,607	827	3.7	Not Available	Not Available	Not Available	Not Available
Jenin		19.34	85	27	580	2,555	811	3.3	Not Available	Not Available	Not Available	Not Available
Dependency Rate												
Less than 1	6.7	23.03	101	32	686	3,023	959	3.4	4.8	143	58	1,717
1-1.99	7	19.5	86	27	555	2,445	776	3.5	3.9	111	47	1,330
2 and More	7.2	18.27	80	26	498	2,195	696	3.7	3.5	97	43	1,160
Main Sources of Income												
Remittances in Cash/Others	6.6	20.12	89	28	543	2,391	758	3.7	4.3	115	51	1,379
Wages and Salaries	7	19.79	87	28	581	2,562	813	3.4	4.0	116	47	1,393
Household Business	7.4	22.24	98	31	672	2,962	940	3.3	4.2	127	50	1,524
Level of Living /b												
Worse-off	7.4	14.14	62	20	457	2,013	639	3.1%	2.7	86	32	1,036
Middle	7	21.17	93	30	598	2,633	835	3.5	4.2	119	51	1,432
Better-off	5.9	31.62	139	44	839	3,696	1,172	3.8	7.5	199	90	2,384
Household Size												
More than 10	12.5	26.16	115	37	791	3,486	1,106	3.3	2.9	88	35	1,062
8-9	8.4	21.23	94	30	668	2,942	933		3.5	111	42	1,333
6-7	6.4	20.5	90	29	592	2,610	828		4.5	129	54	1,553
4-5	4.5	18.96	84	26	510	2,247	713		5.9	158	71	1,901
1-3	2.3	15.25	67	21	368	1,623	515	4.1	9.3	224	111	2,686

a. Medical expenditure includes social health insurance payment;

b: Worse off = food consumption greater than 45 percent total consumption; middle = 30-44 percent total consumption; better off = less than 30 percent of total consumption.

Source: Palestinian Central Bureau of Statistics, 1996. Palestinian Expenditure and Consumption Survey, Ramallah, West Bank, 1996.

ANNEX 13

Annex Table 13.1 : Donor Commitments and Disbursements for 1994 to 1997 by Category of Expenditure

Category	Commitments				Disbursements			
	1994	1995	1996	1997	1994	1995	1996	1997
Transitional Budget Support	1,023	1,602	2,824	2,903	1,023	1,302	2,621	817
Equipment	12,615	4,840	6,730	617	3,361	247	5,085	
In Kind	2,720	5,373	690		2,720	5,651	690	
Public Investment	14,723	17,807	40,144	4,545	12,576	5,485	26,015	600
Technical Assistance	21,011	18,869	9,685	31,607	13,241	19,775	8,950	5,036
Various	3,332	2,567	412	97	375	220	62	
Grand Total	55,424	51,058	60,485	39,769	33,296	32,680	43,423	6,453

Source: MOPIC, 1997.

Annex Table 13.2: Donor Commitments and Disbursements for 1994 to 1997 by Category of Expenditure (in percent)

Category	Commitments				Disbursements			
	1994	1995	1996	1997	1994	1995	1996	1997
Transitional Budget Support	2	3	5	7	3	4	6	13
Equipment	23	9	11	2	10	1	12	0
In Kind	5	11	1	0	8	17	2	0
Public Investment	27	35	66	11	38	17	60	9
Technical Assistance	38	37	16	79	40	61	21	78
Various	6	5	1	0	1	1	0	0
Grand Total	100	100	100	100	100	100	100	100

Source: MOPIC, 1997.

ANNEX 14

Annex Table 14.1: UNRWA Health Expenditures in West Bank and Gaza

Category	1995	1996
Gaza Strip		
Medical Supplies	1,204,243	1,580,589
Lab Supplies	85,031	85,000
Dental Supplies	17,328	16,200
Ahli Arab Hospital	1,354,975	1,102,536
Other Hospitals	215,739	212,057
Staffing	5,346,166	5,009,454
Other Recurrent	2,028,125	1,569,169
Health Education	79,461	8,214
Equipment	1,552,938	421,631
Construction	969,062	712,172
Gaza Strip Total	12,853,068	10,717,022
West Bank		
Qalqilya Hospital		1,012,347
Primary Care		3,297,649
Secondary Care		0
Reimbursements		606,083
Contracts		1,821,911
Capital Spending		1,061,991
Drugs and Disposables		873,613
Salaries		3,789,413
West Bank Total		12,463,007
West Bank and Gaza Total		23,180,029

Source: UNRWA, 1997.

ANNEX 15

Health Worker Wage Rates - UNRWA and Ministry of Health, 1996

UNRWA wage rates, 1997 [66]. A new physician earns on average around $14,657 per year with benefits.

Basic Monthly Salary

Physician	$921
Senior Physician	$1,064
Practical Nurse	$463-$476
Staff Nurse	$532-$580
Technician, Pharmacist	$497
Laborer	$440

Dependency allowance provided up to 7 children:
for 1 - 4 children, $18 per month per child
for 5 - 7 children, $3 per month
spouse, $10 per month

Ministry of Health [67]. Government doctors earn on average around NIS 2,000 per month ($625 per month). Nurses receive between NIS 1,200 - 1,600 per month ($375 - $500 per month), and technicians and administrative staff between NIS 700 - 1,000 per month ($219 - $313 per month). These government wage rates are around two thirds to one half of the wages earned by UNRWA health workers.

Government wages are determined by the PA. Physicians receive up to 100 percent of basic salary in the form of professional allowance, but cannot exceed this level.

---

[66] Source: UNRWA Administrative Office, Gaza City Field Office, 1997.
[67] Source: Ministry of Health, Nablus, Accounting Department, 1997.

ANNEX 16

Annex Table 16.1: West Bank and Gaza: Average Monthly Wage Rates, 1994
4.20 NIS/JD

	Total	Female	Male	Total	Female	Male	Total	Female	Male	Total	Female	Male
	(JD)	(JD)	(JD)	(NIS)	(NIS)	(NIS)	(NIS)	(NIS)	(NIS)			
Total	283	264	284	1,189	1,109	1,193	59	55	60	6.3 %	6.8 %	6.3 %
Illiterate	178	180	177	748	756	743	37	38	37	10.0 %	9.9 %	10.1 %
Secondary and Lower	187	187	243	785	785	1,021	39	39	51	9.5 %	9.5 %	7.3 %
General Secondary Certificate	202	202	281	848	848	1,180	42	42	59	8.8 %	8.8 %	6.4 %
Lower Diploma	281	281	297	1,180	1,180	1,247	59	59	62	6.4 %	6.4 %	6.0 %
BA/BSc	272	272	313	1,142	1,142	1,315	57	57	66	6.6 %	6.6 %	5.7 %
Higher Diploma	305	305	375	1,281	1,281	1,575	64	64	79	5.9 %	5.9 %	4.8 %
MA/MSc	548	548	530	2,302	2,302	2,226	115	115	111	3.3 %	3.3 %	3.4 %
Ph.D.	713	713	815	2,995	2,995	3,423	150	150	171	2.5 %	2.5 %	2.2 %
Unknown	318		318	1,336		1,336	67		67	5.6 %	-	5.6 %

Source: Palestinian Central Bureau of Statistics, Household Survey, 1994.

Annex Table 16.2: Comparison of 5 Percent of Total Income
to Maximum Health Insurance Contribution

	5 % of Total Income (NIS)	Max (NIS)a
Illiterate	37	75
Secondary and Lower	39	75
General Secondary Certificate	42	75
Lower Diploma	59	75
BA/BSc	57	75
Higher Diploma	64	75
MA/MSc	115	75
Ph.D.	150	75

a. Government Health Insurance Premium Ceiling is set at NIS 75.
Source: Palestine Central Bureau of Statistics, Household Survey, 1994.

ANNEX 17

Annex Table 17.1: West Bank and Gaza: Estimation of Government Subsidies for Hospitalization, 1996

	West Bank		Gaza Strip		West Bank and Gaza	
	US$ (thousand)	Percent	US$ (thousand)	Percent	US$ (thousand)	Percent
	actual		estimation/1		estimation/1	
MOH Health Expenditure						
Overseas Treatment	9,231	19	6,476	13	15,707	16
Hospital	21,953	45	22,659	45	44,612	45
Public Health (primary care)	11,073	23	11,429	23	22,502	23
Other	6,258	13	9,511	19	15,769	16
Total	48,515	100	50,075	100	98,590	100
Number of Insured Households	102,723		73,787		176,510	
Cost of Hospitalization per Household, US$ /2	295		386		333	
Contribution per Household	168		181		176	
Copayment per Household	14		26		19	
Subsidy per Household	113		179		138	
Subsidy as Percent of Premium Contribution	67		99		78	

1. For Gaza Strip, the distribution of expenditure between hospital and public health sectors was assumed to be the same as in West Bank.

2. About 10 percent of hospitalization is assumed to be uninsured population. Therefore the total expenditure on hospital for the insured population was reduced by 10 percent.

Source: Ministry of Health, World Bank Staff Estimates.

Appendix 11: REPRODUCTIVE HEALTH

INTRODUCTION

Women's health status in the West Bank and Gaza (WBG) has been relatively good in comparison with other similar level of economies and countries in the Middle East and North Africa region (Table A 11.1). This is largely owing to the successful primary health care programs and relatively high educational level of women in the WBG. The Ministry of Health (MOH) of Palestinian Authority (PA), UNRWA and NGOs have been providing maternal and child health (MCH) services free of charge. Although family planning services are provided by NGOs, UNRWA, and the MOH, fertility in the WBG is still one of the highest in the world.

The concept of reproductive health has been accepted world wide as the result of two consequent international conferences: International Conference for Population and Development, Cairo 1994; and the Fourth International Conference on Women, Beijing 1995. However, reproductive health is still a new concept for Palestinian women. In addition, there are some gaps between genders in terms of access to health services. In the past one and half year, the MOH, in collaboration with international agencies, has been proceeding with a comprehensive approach for attaining reproductive health.

Table A 11.1: Selected Health and Social Indicators for the West Band and Gaza and Selected Middle Eastern Countries (Most recent estimates from 1993 to 1996)

		West Bank and Gaza	West Bank	Gaza Strip	Jordan	Egypt	Lebanon	Tunisia	Turkey	Lower Middle Income Economies	Israel
GNP per Capita in US$		1,710	2,359	1,199	1,510	790	2,660	1,820	2,780	1,090	15,920
Population (million)		2.5	1.6	0.9	4.2	57.8	4.0	9.0	61.1	-	5.5
Life Expectancy at Birth (year)	Female	74	-	-	72	64	70	70	69	65	78
	Male	70	-	-	68	61	67	68	64		75
Infant Mortality Rate (per 1,000 live births)		28	25	32	34	57	32	40	49	60	8
Maternal Mortality Ratio (per 100,000 live births)		70	-	-	45	170	300	139	183	-	7
Total Fertility Rate		6.9	6.2[a]	7.4[a]	4.6	3.5	2.9	3.0	2.7	3.1	2.4
Contraceptive Prevalence Rate (percent) (Modern Methods)		45 (31)	50 (34)	34 (24)	35 (27)	48 (45)	-	60 (52)	63 (35)	-	-
Annual Population Growth Rate (percent)		3.7	3.5	4.2	3.6	1.9	1.9	1.8	1.6	1.6	2.7
Adult Literacy Rate (percent)	Female	84	90	76	79	39	90	55	72	61	93
	Male				93	64	95	79	92	79	97

a. The MOH's figures in 1996 are 6.0 in West Bank and 6.02 in Gaza Strip.
Sources: Palestinian Central Bureau of Statistics 1996; Health Nutrition and Population Sector Strategy, World Development Report, Hashemite Kingdom of Jordan Health Sector Study, the World Bank, 1997; The State of the World's Children, UNICEF, 1998.

PRESENT REPRODUCTIVE HEALTH SITUATION

Maternal Health

As shown by indicators in Table A 11.1, maternal health status in the WBG is relatively good. Maternal mortality ratio (MMR) in average is about 70 per 100,000 live births while infant mortality rate (IMR) is 28 per 1,000 live births and low birth weight newborns only six percent[68]. MMR in West Bank is higher than that in Gaza Strip although total fertility rate (TFR) is comparatively higher in Gaza Strip. This is probably due to the difficult access to emergency referral services in some areas of West Bank.

Primary health care facilities run by the MOH, UNRWA, NGOs and the private sector provide antenatal care, which usually includes checking blood pressure and anemia and providing tetanus toxoid immunization. About 80 percent pregnant women receive antenatal care at least once; 42 percent receive more than four times. Normal antenatal care is provided by specialists, general physicians, midwives or nurses, while high risk cases are refereed to the hospitals or high risk clinics where specialists are available, and encouraged to deliver in hospitals. Common complications are: anemia, diabetes, hypertension, pre-eclampsia and bleeding. According to the recent reproductive health survey in West Bank, 89 percent of women receive antenatal care at private clinics and NGO facilities[69].

Compared to antenatal care, most women do not routinely receive postnatal care. Although hospitals recommend at least 8 to 48 hours post partum admission, most women discharge a few hours after the delivery. Only 20 percent women receive post-natal check-up, in many cases when they bring their babies for medical consultation. Some clinics are trying to start postnatal home visit by nurses or midwives, however, it is still difficult because of staffing and budgetary constraint. Breast feeding is encouraged during postnatal care and at well-baby clinic during growth monitoring. About 96 percent of infants are breastfed, but about seven percent are weaned within the first three months.

Most deliveries are attended by professionals at the public and private hospitals. In Gaza Strip, 61 percent of deliveries take place at public and UNRWA hospitals and health centers, nine percent in NGO and private hospitals, 26 percent at private clinics, and four percent at home. In West Bank, 54 percent of delivery take place at public and UNRWA hospitals and health centers, 30 percent in NGO and private hospitals, three percent at private clinics, and 13 percent at home. About half of home deliveries are attended by traditional birth attendants (TBAs), relatives or friends. There are regional variations: 30 percent of deliveries in Hebron district are taken place at home, of which two thirds (about 20 percent of total deliveries) are attended by TBAs; almost all the home deliveries in Tulkarm and Salfit districts, which reach 28 percent of total deliveries, are attended by TBAs. Private maternity hospitals are remarkably increasing in urban areas as seen by more deliveries taking place in the private sector hospitals than public hospitals in Bethlehem and Qalquilya districts.

Since the private hospitals and clinics, as well as UNRWA health centers, usually handle only normal or low risk cases, obstetric emergencies and high risk cases are usually refereed to

---

[68] Palestinian Central Bureau of Statistics 1996.

[69] Ismail and Shahin: Family planning and women's reproductive health survey. Planning and Research Center, Jerusalem (1996).

the MOH hospitals where operation and blood transfusion can be done. Palestine Red Crescent Society (PRCS) also runs first referral level maternity hospitals in West Bank. The public sector is responsible for managing difficult cases but efficient emergency referral is sometimes difficult because of political conditions such as frequent closures[70].

Induced abortion is approved only by medical reasons according to Islamic regulations, although it is not clear that what medical reasons can be applied. For example, some physicians say that abortion can be applied in case the woman's health (not life) is at risk or the fetus has genetic abnormality. It is not known how often and by whom illicit abortion takes place.

Table A 11.2: Health Care Facilities (1997)

		Health Centers and Clinics	MCH Centers and Clinics	Hospitals + Maternity Hospitals
Ministry of Health	West Bank	178	9	8
	Gaza Strip	31	(24)[a]	5
UNRWA	West Bank	34	0	1
	Gaza Strip	12	6	0
Nongovernmental Organizations/ Private	West Bank	340	9	7 + 7
	Gaza Strip	31	(20)[a]	3 + 2
Total	West Bank	552	18	16 + 7
	Gaza Strip	74	6 (+ 44)	8 + 2
	Total	626	24 (+ 44)	33

a. MCH centers integrated in health centers.
Sources: Ministry of Health 1997; The Status of Health in Palestine Annual Report 1996; WHO 1996.

Table A 11.3: Human Resources in Health

			Physicians	Nurses	Total (include technicians, administrators, etc.)
MOH (1996)	Hospitals	West Bank	339	769	1,846
		Gaza Strip	436	707	1,761
	Public Health	West Bank	136	321	885
		Gaza Strip	191	295	1,346
		Total	1,102	2,092	5,838
UNRWA Health Sector (1995)		West Bank	52	176	298
		Gaza Strip	57	184	308
		Total	109	360	606
NGO Primary Health (1993)		West Bank	392	214	810
		Gaza Strip	129	124	349
		Total	521	338	1,159

Sources: The Status of Health in Palestine Annual Report 1996; WHO 1996; Gaza Health Services Research Center 1996; Palestinian Ministry of Health Nablus 1996; UNRWA 1996 Annual Report of the Department of Health 1995; Planning and Research Center 1994.

Family Planning

[70] The MOH reported that at least four deliveries were taken place at the checkpoints in West Bank during the closure in September 1997. One of the four newborns died three days later.

Although primary health care services have covered most of the population in the WBG and succeeded in decreasing IMR, family planning services still remain insufficient. The MOH estimated TFR in 1996 at 6.02 in Gaza Strip and 6.0 in West Bank. The acceptance of family planning was culturally and politically difficult in the past, especially during the period of *intifada*. However, the recent political change and economic stagnation have increased the demand of family planning dramatically. Contraceptive prevalence rate has reached 45 percent in a recent study in West Bank[71]. Leaders of religious groups endorse family planning as not offensive against religious belief.

NGOs and private sectors have been playing major roles in family planning services. For example, Jordanian Family Planning and Protection Association was established in Jerusalem as early as 1963 and was the first Arab world establishment of International Planned Parenthood Federation (IPPF). After the Israeli occupation in 1967, Palestinian Family Planning and Protection Association (PFPPA) was split from the Jordanian association. The Palestinian association not only provides family planning services through its own clinics, but also provides contraceptives and technical assistance to other local NGOs. The association is also active in information, education and communication (IEC) programs such as promoting awareness among youths. UNRWA has been providing family planning services as part of its primary health care services since 1990. The MOH started to provide family planning services in 1994.

The most popular modern contraceptive method is IUD (Figure A 11.1,2) and is inserted by doctors at private clinics, female doctors at family planning units of the public health centers, and trained nurses at UNRWA and NGO clinics. Pills, condoms and spermicides are also used; injections are recently used in the public health facilities, but not in UNRWA clinics following Jordanian regulation[72]. Norplant, tubal ligation and vasectomy are not approved as contraceptive methods, although tubal ligation is sometimes performed during Cesarean section or by laparoscopy. More than 60 percent of modern contraceptive services are provided by the private sector. About one fourths of pills and condoms are distributed by private pharmacies.

Recent health survey in West Bank shows that 45 percent of women are currently using contraceptives and 30 percent use modern methods[73]. About half of non-users wish to use contraceptives in near future. Contraceptives are most popular among women who already have completed the desired number of children, usually including at least two boys. Although about 80 percent of ever-users answered that birth spacing is the main reason for starting to use contraceptives, young women, particularly under 20 years old, are reluctant to use contraceptives for birth spacing. The main reasons of non-use or discontinuation are: want children, husband objection, social pressure and side effect (Table A 11.4). More counseling and advocacy, especially among males, are needed.

---

[71] Ismail and Shahin: Family planning and women's reproductive health survey. Planning and Research Center, Jerusalem (1996). The MOH estimates contraceptive prevalence rate in Gaza Strip at 30 - 32 percent in 1997.

[72] The ratio of the purpose of visit to the nine MOH clinics in Gaza Strip from January to April 1997 (total 5,279 visits) were: 30 percent for pills; 10 percent for IUD insertion; 19 percent for condom; 3 percent for spermicides; 3 percent for injection; and 2 percent for IUD extraction.

[73] Ismail and Shahin: Family planning and women's reproductive health survey. Planning and Research Center, Jerusalem (1996).

Table A 11.4: Reasons for Non-use and Discontinuation of Contraceptives

Reasons for Non-use	Percent	Reasons for Discontinuation	Percent
Menopause	44	Want Children	29
Husband Objection	18	Social Pressure	20
Opposing Family Planning	13	Side Effect	17
Fear Of Side Effect	11	Health Concern	6
Religious Belief	7	Pregnant During Using Contraceptives	6
Inconvenient	4	Not Sexually Active	4

Source: The health survey in the West Bank and Gaza Strip. Palestinian Central Bureau of Statistics (1997); Shurbasi, A. Current practices of contraceptive use at MCH center, Gaza field. UNRWA, Gaza (1995).

Figure A 11.1: Contraceptive Practice among Refugee Mothers in Gaza Strip

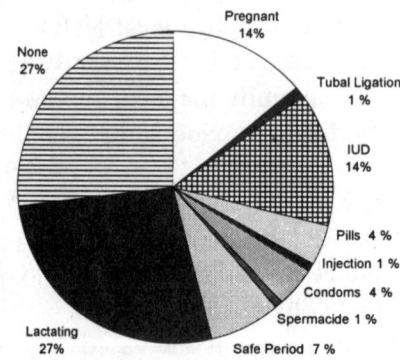

Source: Shurbasi, A. <u>Current Practices of Contraceptive Use at MCH Center, Gaza Field</u>. UNRWA, Gaza (1995).

Figure A 11.2: Contraceptive Practice among Married Women in West Bank

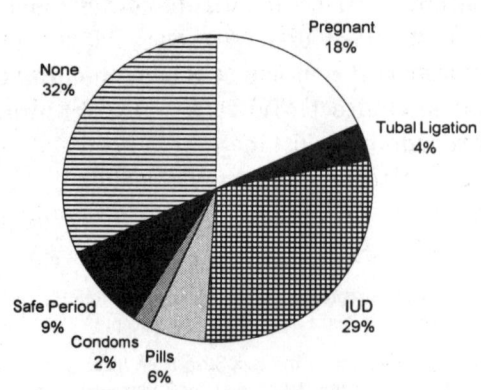

Source: <u>Family Planning and Women's Reproductive Health Survey</u>. Planning and Research Center (1996).

Sexual Transmitted Diseases

It is believed that incidence of sexual transmitted diseases (STD) is low in the WBG. Only four gonorrhea cases and no syphilis case were reported to the MOH in 1996. Physicians in public hospitals say that they never encounter syphilis or gonorrhea, but do find quite a few cases of minor infection caused by trichomonas or candida. STD surveillance system has not been reliable enough. Because of lack of adequate counseling services and shortage of female doctors, women are often reluctant to seek care even they have symptom of STD.

Donor blood is routinely screened for hepatitis B (HB) but not for VDRL, while HIV testing is done only for suspected cases. In 1996, 1,178 HB carriers and 114 HB cases, 73 hepatitis C carriers and one case were reported. In 1996, among tested donor samples in the blood banks of MOH hospital in West Bank, HB antigen positive cases were 477 out of 16,826 samples, and hepatitis C positive cases were 50 out of 14,249 samples. HB antigen positive cases were four to five percent among 17,424 samples tested at the Central Laboratory in Gaza Strip in 1996 and hepatitis C positive cases were one to two percent among 10,150 samples. Two positive VDRLs found among 1,222 samples were confirmed as false positive at an Israeli referral laboratory. Newborns are now routinely vaccinated against HB.

During 1987-1993, 24 AIDS cases were reported among Palestinians in WBG and Jerusalem. Seven cases were adult women while two were infants. Six cases were transmitted heterosexually, four homosexually, and six through blood transfusion and blood products. Among 15,498 donor samples tested in the blood banks at MOH hospitals in West Bank in 1996, two samples were found HIV positive. Among the 12,439 samples tested at the Central Laboratory in Gaza Strip in 1996, only one was HIV positive and the patient died in two weeks. In 1994, the Laboratory found an HIV positive pregnant woman, whose infant was also infected. Both mother and child eventually died of AIDS. Since only suspected cases are tested, the accurate HIV positive rate is not yet known.

Cancers in Women

About one tenths of deaths are caused by cancer, which is the third leading cause of death among adults. Since cancer screening programs do not exist and only limited number of facilities have pathology units, accurate cancer incidences among women have not been determined yet. According to the 1994 study, mammary cancer comprised 28.5 percent, uterine corpus cancer 5.5 percent, uterine cervical cancer 3.1 percent, and ovarian cancer 4.1 percent of the 3,435 female cancer cases included in the study. The incidence of uterine cervical cancer appeared to be relatively low among Palestinian women, which may relate to their life style. Mammary and uterine cancer incidences increase dramatically after 45 years of age (Table A 11.5). This suggests that cancer prevention programs should target menopausal and post menopausal women at first.

Table A 11.5: Age Distribution of Mammary, Uterine and Ovarian Cancer Cases

	Number of Cases	Age Distribution (years)			
		- 25	25 - 35	35 - 45	46 -
Mammary Cancer	980	10	93	249	628
Uterine Corps Cancer	189	0	3	22	164
Uterine Cervical Cancer	107	1	13	23	70
Ovarian Cancer	140	27	20	29	64
Total	1,416	38	129	323	926
Rate (percent)	100	2.7	9.1	22.8	65.4

Source: Abdeen, Z. and Barghuthy, F. Palestinian cancer statistics, seventeen years of cancer incidence, 1976-1992. Data Bank and Health Related Research Center, Arab College of Medical Professions, Al-Quds University (1994).

Adolescent Health

Early marriage is still common among Palestinian girls. Currently, girls are allowed to marry at 16 years of age, following Islamic regulations that allow marriage when girls become physically and mentally matured. However, quite a few number of girls get married even at the age of 14 or 15 years. Early marriage is likely to cause high risk pregnancies, high fertility and low education attainment. Women Health and Development Administration of the MOH, Directorate of Gender Planning and Development of the Ministry of Planning and International Cooperation (MOPIC), UNRWA, and NGOs are advocating health and economic benefits of later marriage. Marriage between cousins or relatives are common and result in relatively high incidences of genetic or inherited disorders such as thalasemia.

UNRWA's school health program is targeted to ninth grade girls, many of whom are about to marry. UNRWA nurses visit schools and teach family health classes. The MOH's Health Education Department also conducts school health programs and youth programs in Gaza Strip. However, health education and counseling regarding sexuality among youths are still very limited. Some of NGOs' IEC programs are targeting youth groups, which include training of youth peer counselors. It is difficult for unmarried youth to access family planning services.

Women's Health During and Post Menopause

Nearly half of Palestinian female population is under 15 years old, reproductive age women are 43 percent of female population and only 10 percent is older than 49 years old. Until now, very little is known about women's health during and post menopause. Particular programs targeting elder women have not been developed.

Infertility

Although having children is considered to be of social value to women, accurate rate and cause of infertility is not yet known. The rate of infertility among Palestinian couples is estimated to be at the same level as that in developed countries. According to the 1996 reproductive health survey in West Bank, seven percent of women have never been pregnant as yet, and 28 percent women wanted to be pregnant as soon as possible. Since women are expected to be pregnant immediately after getting married, it is not unusual that women visit physicians seek treatment of infertility only two or three months after marriage. A private in vitro fertilization clinic has opened in Nablus, suggesting that there are women who desperately want to get pregnant. Infertility counseling and treatment integrated with other reproductive health services, standard protocol for infertility treatment, and technical and ethical regulation for applying advanced reproductive technique have to be established urgently[74].

Mental health and violence against women

Due to the difficult social and economic situation and restricted social mobility, many women are said to be suffering from mental disorders such as depression. Besides the violence caused by political turmoil, women are also exposed to various degrees of domestic violence. For example one woman in Gaza Strip and another in West Bank were killed in a month by their male family members due to "disgrace of the family honor." Constant threat by domestic violence affects women's mental condition to a large extent. However, female genital mutilation is not practiced among Palestinian women, unlike neighboring Egypt.

NEW APPROACHES AND CHALLENGES FOR COMPREHENSIVE REPRODUCTIVE HEALTH SERVICES

PA is giving serious attention to promote women's health and has emphasized equality and non-discrimination in public rights of men and women in the "Palestinian Declaration of Independence." Directorate of Gender Planning and Development, MOPIC, advocates various women's issues, prepares the Palestinian National Plan of Action for the Advancement of Women and coordinates inter-ministerial committee for women's development.

Women's Health and Development Administration was established in the MOH one and half year ago. Following the Strategic Plan for Women Health and Development in Palestine, the administration is promoting a comprehensive approach for reproductive health. Receiving three year financial support of ECU 4.5 million from European Commission (EC), the MOH is building family planning units in the existing health facilities and providing training for nurses and doctors. Up to 15 health centers in West Bank are to be upgraded, and eight MOH health centers and three NGO clinics in Gaza Strip currently provide family planning services. IPPF, through PFPPA, has also supported to provide family planing services in five MOH health centers. EC and IPPF support provision of contraceptives, too. Recently UNFPA proposed technical and financial support of US $1.2 million over the next five years.

Human resource development is vital for providing comprehensive reproductive health services. Since family planning, STD management and other reproductive health services are to be integrated into the existing primary health care services, health professionals need to be trained both technically and conceptually. To encourage women for seeking care, doctors and nurses need to develop counseling skills and qualified female service providers need to be increased.

---

[74] Recently the MOH started to prepare a standard protocol for infertility treatment in West Bank, that emphasize counseling and prevention of pelvic inflammatory diseases.

RECOMMENDATIONS FOR THE MEDIUM TERM STRATEGY AND IMMEDIATE INTERVENTIONS

Public and Private Role

Considering the current heavy involvement of the private sector in providing reproductive health services, the roles of public and private sectors need to be defined in the medium term. The MOH is responsible for establishing legal framework to secure efficient provision of reproductive health services and for monitoring the quality of services and supervising health professionals. The MOH also need to establish financing and payment mechanism for both public and private sectors for sustaining reproductive health services and securing access to services. On the other hand, the MOH will be able to hand over the provision of family planning services to the NGO and private sector, when public becomes well aware of the benefit and access to the services are secured. Most low risk maternal care services can also be provided by the NGO and private sector under the MOH's quality monitoring.

In addition to regulation and monitoring, the MOH hospitals have responsibility to handle obstetric emergencies and difficult cases. An efficient referral system needs to be established in the medium term. Recently, the MOH designated PRCS to provide ambulance services in the WBG. The ambulance services will possibly connect primary health care services provided mainly by the private sector, to the referral services mainly provided by the public sector. Primary health care personnel need to be further trained for the selection of cases and timing of referral. Political issues which obstruct emergency transportation may remain for an uncertain period of time.

Upgraded Preventive Care

Although preventive care for women's health in the WBG is relatively good, more efforts are needed to raise public awareness of promoting reproductive health. The following are examples which can be started immediately once health personnel are trained:

- nutritional education to prevent complications during pregnancy, such as hypertension and diabetes;
- increased postnatal care coverage at clinics, as well as by home visits;
- promotion of birth spacing among young women[75];
- raising husbands' awareness of family planning[76];
- health education including sexuality and reproductive health for male and female youths;
- premarriage counseling including knowledge of genetic diseases;
- improved counseling services for family planning, STD, infertility and mental health;

Before starting new interventions, it is necessary to have accurate figures of prevalence and incidence. For example, STD is obviously under-reported and it is necessary to establish a surveillance system which is integrated to the ongoing health information system development. Cancer screening programs have not been undertaken as yet. Taking into account the

---

[75] The MOH has already started to implement this recommendation.

[76] The MOH has started awareness programs targeting ninth grade school children, young men, husbands, and old women who often make decisions in households.

population's age structure and disease pattern, possible cancer screening programs have to be carefully planned and prioritized after extensive cost-benefit analyses.

Interventions targeted to underprivileged areas

Despite a relatively small population concentrate in small areas, there are some regional differences in terms of access and attitude to health care services. Access to the family planning services and advocation of the benefit, especially to males, needs to be strengthened in Gaza Strip. Maternal care services need to be improved in particular districts in West Bank. Some of the public facilities for deliveries need to be rehabilitated.

Cost of reproductive health interventions

Cost of providing reproductive health care in the WBG, comprising of benefits such as maternal care, obstetric and neonatal complications, management of incomplete abortion, treatment of STD and family planning services, is estimated at US$6.6 million annually. This assumes that 100 percent of pregnancies will be provided with maternal care and that family planning services can be extended to at least 50 percent of all married women in the reproductive age group. Prevalence of STD and of different complications of pregnancy have been taken into account when estimating the cost required for their management.

Table A 11.6 shows the cost of different interventions by level of health care. It is assumed that about 50 percent of women will have contact with clinics, 40 percent including referrals will be utilizing comprehensive health centers and 10 percent will have contact with hospitals. Cost per client at the clinic is minimal at US$7.5 per client with provision of only basic maternity care, STD and family planning services; US$22.6 at comprehensive centers where management of some complicated cases will also done; and is US$64.5 at hospitals. Calculations assume that no new construction is done and share of overhead costs such as maintenance, salaries, equipment, etc. are assigned to the reproductive health package.

Table A 11.6: Summary of Cost by Service Levels

	Cost (US$)	Share (percent)	Per Client (US$)	Per Capita (US$)	Per Birth (US$)
Clinic	1,278,256	19.4	7.45	0.56	-
Comprehensive Health Center	3,107,220	47.1	22.64	1.36	-
Hospital	2,214,654	33.6	64.54	0.97	-
Total	6,600,630	100.0		2.90	65.80

Source: World Bank staff estimates.

As described previously, the coverage of maternal care and other basic primary health care services in the WBG is relatively high. In addition, the MOH, in collaboration with donor agencies, has already started to upgrade reproductive health services including family planning services. Therefore if we assume that required staff and equipment is to a great extent present in most facilities, the cost estimated would be reduced by more than two thirds to US$1.9 million. This includes training for physicians, nurses and midwives; incentives for their additional workload; and recurrent costs and is the equivalent of US$19 per birth or $0.83 per capita.

CONCLUSION

Comprehensive approach for reproductive health service has started in the WBG. The MOH, in collaboration with international agencies and NGOs, is taking measures steadily for improving women's health. Considering relatively high education level among women, it is expected to achieve major progress in near future. After the transitional stage, the role of the MOH needs to be re-defined for better utilization of resources and promotion of public and private partnership.

RESOURCE PERSONS

Dr. Munzer Sharif, Deputy Minister, Ministry of Health

Dr. Dina Abu-Sha'ban, Director of Women Health and Development Administration, Gaza, Ministry of Health

Dr. Souzan Abdu, Director of Women Health and Development Administration, Nablus, West Bank, Ministry of Health

Dr. Faten El-Hammami, Director of Family Planning, Gaza, Ministry of Health

Dr. Randa El-Khodary, Director, Central Laboratory, Gaza, Ministry of Health

Ms. Zahira Kamal, General Director, Directorate of Gender Planning and Development, Ministry of Planning and International Cooperation

Dr. Amna Shurbasi, Field Family Health Officer, UNRWA Field Office, Gaza

Ms. Joyce Ajlouny, National Programme Officer, UNFPA

Ms. Monica Awad, Senior Health Assistant, UNICEF

Ms. Battina Musheidt, European Commission Technical Assistance Office

Mr. Haidar Husseini, Secretary General
Ms. Dima Aweidah-Nashashibi, Executive Director
Mr. Ziad Yaish, IEC Officer
Palestinian Family Planning and Protection Association, Executive Office, Jerusalem

Mr. Younis N. Al-Khatib, General Director
Dr. Izzat N. Ayoub, Emergency Medical Services Department
Palestine Red Crescent Society

REFERENCES

Women Health and Development Administration, Ministry of Health: Strategic plan for women health and development in Palestine. (1995).

Women Health and Development Administration, Ministry of Health: Achievement of women's health and development administration for 1996. (1997).

Directorate of Gender Planning and Development, Ministry of Planning and International Cooperation: Directorate of gender planning and development, a concept paper, mission and conceptual framework. (1996).

Health Research and Planning Directorate, Statistics and Information Department, Ministry of Health: The Status of Health in Palestine Annual Report 1996. (1997)

Statistics and Information Department, Ministry of Health: Health statistics, West Bank districts. (1996).

National Health Plan Commission: The national health plan for the Palestinian people, objectives and strategies. Planning and Research Center, Jerusalem (1994).

Palestinian Central Bureau of Statistics: The health survey in the West Bank and Gaza Strip, main findings. (1997).

Ismail, N., and Shahin, M.: Family planning and women's reproductive health survey. Planning and Research Center, Jerusalem (1996).

Stephenson, P.: The health of Palestinian women in the West Bank and Gaza Strip, problems and priorities - resources and opportunities. UNICEF, Jerusalem (1996).

UNFPA: Programme of assistance to the Palestinian people in Gaza and West Bank. (1996).

United Nations General Assembly Official Records - Fifty-first Session: Report of the Commissioner-General of the United Nations Relief and Works Agency for Palestine Refugees in the Near East, 1 July 1995 - 30 June 1996. United Nations, New York (1996).

Shurbasi, A.: Current practices of contraceptive use at MCH center, Gaza field. UNRWA Field Office, Gaza (1995).

Palestinian Family Planning and Protection Association, International Planned Parenthood Federation Arab World Region, Palestinian Red Crescent Society, and European Commission: The Palestinian conference on population and family planning, final statement and recommendations, Palestine Hospital, Cairo. (1994).

Barghouthi, M. and Lennock, J. Health in Palestine: Potential and Challenges. Palestine Economic Policy Research Institute (MAS). (1997)

Abdeen, Z. and Barghuthy, F. Palestinian cancer statistics, seventeen years of cancer incidence, 1976-1992. Data Bank and Health Related Research Center, Arab College of Medical Professions, Al-Quds University (1994).

Abdeen, Z. and Barghuthy, F. Acquired immunodeficiency syndrome (AIDS), questions and answers. Data Bank and Health Related Research Center, Arab College of Medical Professions, Al-Quds University (1994).

Appendix 12: THE PHARMACEUTICAL SECTOR

BACKGROUND

This working paper is part of the Health Sector Study commissioned by the Ministry of Health (MOH), the World Health Organization (WHO) and the World Bank. The pharmaceutical sector study and other sub-sector studies were carried out from May 9 to 22, 1997. It included visits to the MOH, hospitals, health centers, pharmaceutical wholesalers, factories, retail pharmacies, and numerous NGO and UN organizations involved in health care in the West Bank and Gaza (WBG). The study draws upon work done in 1993 by UNICEF, and on a WHO supported analysis of the drugs situation conducted by the MOH in 1997. Available data on the drug sector has been reviewed.

The study is based primarily on analysis of data. Observations on the working of the sector and detailed interviews with numerous stakeholders were undertaken to confirm data and solicit opinions on the achievements. It considers problems and possible future strategies for improvements in the pharmaceutical sector in support of an improved quality of care in the WBG. Though some data and figures are difficult to validate, however most figures are believed to be accurate within a range of plus or minus 10 percent. Given the transitional situation in the WBG, the analysis and recommendations can quite safely be made even with such uncertainty.

EXECUTIVE SUMMARY

Major Issues

The annual cost of drugs to the individual and society is high and increasing. The per capita consumption is US$21 - 29, and in total US$47 - 67 million. The 1997 projected budget for drugs and consumables is 30 percent of total MOH expenditure, up from 28 percent in 1996. The drug costs are also high when compared to countries at the same level of socio-economic development. About 10 drugs, often very sophisticated ones, consume about 25 percent of the annual drug budget.

There is no national drug policy and a very antiquated drug legislation. These factors are a major impediment to the rational and cost-effective development of the pharmaceutical sector.

There are eight pharmaceutical companies, while a new plant is under construction. They produce about 50 percent of total consumption. Although none of the factories are producing according to good manufacturing standards, they are quite successful in winning MOH tenders. The relatively low prices offered to the MOH are offset by much higher prices in the private sector. Plant utilization is low, with even those at higher utilization operating at perhaps two to three times greater costs than comparable factories in other countries. Israeli restrictions on importation from abroad provides a shield for the industry in terms of prices, but also results in higher prices in both the public and private sectors. The industry produces many combination products, i.e. with two or more active ingredients. These products are not generally recommended. Existing drug formulations are copied locally and marketed as branded generics

There may be as many as 4,000 different drugs on the market. This is very high compared to countries with a rational drug policy. There is a trend towards limited drug lists, but a national essential drug list is still in draft form. Many NGOs and UNRWA use such essential drug lists, and MOH tenders for only about 600 different drugs under generic names.

The pharmaceutical sector administration has only been in existence for about two years. It is suffering from severe resource constraints in terms of qualified staff, equipment, computers and transportation, as well as access to knowledge of modern drug administration.

There is good availability of drugs. However, drug consumption is very much demand and consumption driven, rather than based on medical needs and morbidity statistics.

Drug prices are very high in the private sector. MOH is reasonably successful in securing prices for most drugs which are not much higher than average international prices. However, UNRWA's prices are consistently lower. The Israeli requirement that drugs must be registered in Israel is a hindrance to the import of low-cost generics into WBG. Households spend about US$168 per year on drugs and vitamins, which is equivalent to 50 percent of their total health budget. In 1996, MOH's budget for drugs, funded from general revenue, was US$17.5 million. Both the NIS 3 paid per drug item by patients in MOH facilities and the 17 percent VAT in private pharmacies, revert to the Ministry of Finance.

There is widespread overprescription and polypharmacy, particularly of antibiotics, injections and combination products. The absence of standard treatment protocols makes it difficult to monitor and control prescription practices. Doctors in private practice rely primarily on expensive branded products and the present drug law does not allow for generic substitution.

There are about 560 private pharmacies which is a high figure considering the small size of the population and the relatively short distances. The present pharmacy law and new regulations stipulate that pharmacies must be 100 meters or more apart but cannot limit the number of pharmacies when applicants meet the legal requirements. Many pharmacy owners have a hard time running a profitable business.

Framework for Reform

While the issue of availability of drugs in most facilities seems to have been solved, there is plenty of scope for reform of the pharmaceutical sector. The major objectives for reform are:

- Cost containment

- The rational use of drugs

There is abundant international experience in reforming the pharmaceutical sector, in particular the public sector. Such experience and "best practices" from other countries should be carefully reviewed with a view to determining how they can best be used in the WBG.

Any major reform is likely to provoke resistance, if not outright protests. The presence of numerous stakeholders and much vested interest must be considered in the planning of extensive reforms.

Experience has shown that major reform elements should not only be carefully planned but also gradually introduced. Nearly all elements of the present drug sector should be made the subject of detailed reviews with changes carefully planned and implemented. There is already a reasonable volume of studies and research, and more studies are under way. This seems to provide sufficient material for reform activities to start soon.

The reform process should be carefully designed by experts with relevant country experience. WHO and the World Bank may be relied upon to identify expertise for providing technical support to MOH staff. An important element is to involve as many stakeholders as possible in the process. The study's recommendations are therefore listed in terms of how they can be most easily implemented.

While there is no blueprint for reform, the new edition of Managing Drugs Supply (MSH with WHO, 1997) can serve as a useful tool for reform and not least for teaching and training of all health staff involved in the management of drugs and vaccines.

Conclusions and Recommendations

This study concludes that MOH has achieved a major success, under difficult circumstances, in securing the regular availability of drugs and vaccines. However, availability has been achieved at a high cost.

There are too many drugs in the sector and prices in the private sector are very high. The domestic industry provides a large share of the annual consumption, but does not operate efficiently in terms of quality and price.

Consumption is too driven by past consumption and patients' demand for drugs. There are also too many private pharmacies in operation. Restrictions on the part of Israel with regard to drug registration influence the WBG drug market, not least in terms of branded products and resulting high prices.

The study also concludes that there is considerable scope for reform of the health sector to contain costs and to rationalize the use of drugs.

The study makes the following major recommendations:

- Implement a national essential drugs list with standard treatment protocols;

- Seek lifting of Israeli drug registration requirements;

- Shift estimation of drug requirements to morbidity and service statistics;

- Improve drug price intelligence for better procurement prices;

- Introduce generic substitution;

- Draft a National Drug Policy and a modern drug legislation.

INTRODUCTION

In 1996, the 2.3 million residents of the WBG consumed drugs and vaccines worth a total cost of at least $47 million, or $21 per person. Due to considerable uncertainly about the size of the private sector, this estimate may be significantly low. Some sources indicate that private sector provision may be much more substantial, estimating total annual drug consumption at $67 million, or $29 per person. In comparison, Israeli consumption was $53 in 1996 and Jordanian $36 in 1995 (up from $21 in 1994). In Egypt, annual drug consumption is about $15 per capita and further declining.

Drugs and vaccines are provided from multiple sources, including the MOH (37 percent), NGOs (17 percent), UNRWA (4 percent), UNICEF (vaccines), WHO (polio-vaccine), other UN and bilateral donations, and the private pharmacy sector (42 percent). Drugs are procured from eight domestic manufacturers, from Israeli factories and from abroad through agents and wholesalers. While most donations are in cash to finance local procurement of domestic or imported drugs, some are made in kind.

Availability of drugs and vaccines to cover the needs of the health services and the population has been and continues to be good and regular. Drugs not available in a given sub-sector can normally be obtained from another source, often from a private pharmacy. This is a major achievement for the Palestinian Authority (PA) and the MOH, as very few countries have gone through a period of rapid transition and turmoil without experiencing severe shortages of even vital drugs.

Despite good availability, there are disparities and inequities in access. While refugees, insured people, and registered social welfare patients have access to free or subsidized drugs, uninsured and poorer patients frequently have access only to expensive pharmacy drugs. Because fees for subsidized outpatient department (OPD) drugs are low, better off patients may get normally expensive drugs at very low cost to themselves. However, the General Administration of Pharmacy's ability to cope with the drug situation augurs well for future improvements in the supply of pharmaceuticals.

Good availability has also not been without cost. In 1996 the total cost of drugs and disposables was about 1.9 percent of GDP. In 1997, expenditures for drugs and disposable supplies are projected at 32.5 percent of total MOH expenditures, up from 28.6 percent in 1996 and 21.5 percent in 1995. This is the fastest growth of any single line item in the budget and is not sustainable in the long run.

In 1996 the top 10 drugs consumed about 25 percent of MOH's drug budget. These drugs are mostly expensive remedies for immunosuppression, hematological and hormonal disorders, and latest generation antibiotics. Some are not on WHO's list of essential drugs. High costs per patient and the prospect of increasing demand for treatment of chronic conditions as the epidemiological transition unfolds call for increased attention to the cost of procurement, selection of and rational use of drugs. The current situation presents many challenges as well as multiple options for improving the drugs situation now and in the future. Proven approaches to cost-containment in the supply of pharmaceuticals exist. A strategy to reduce cost without negative medical results would be a priority in halting cost escalation and eventually reducing the total cost of drugs to the population.

NATIONAL DRUG POLICY AND LEGISLATION

There is no national drug policy (NDP). Lack of time, pressing daily problems and lack of resources have prevented the MOH from developing such a policy. However, plans for an NDP have been drawn up in collaboration with WHO's Drug Action Program. The current legislative framework is severely outdated: the West Bank follows the Jordanian Pharmaceutical Association Law of 1957 while Gaza Strip follows the Egyptian Public Health Law of 1956. These laws deal primarily with retail pharmacy practice and are unsuitable to cover or facilitate development of a modern pharmaceutical sector.

The sector is governed less by these laws than by a combination of past practices, MOH decrees and guidelines, and international rules for Good Manufacturing Practice (GMP). Sector management is still somewhat influenced by the former Israeli administration, as registration is not yet completely under Palestinian control. The Israeli requirement that all drugs imported into WBG be registered in Israel both presents a barrier to entry for many low–cost generic manufacturers, and provides a captive market for higher priced Israeli products. At the same time, Israel does not register products produced in the West Bank or registered with the Palestinian authorities.

The lack of clear NDP objectives and strategies, supported by modern drug legislation and ministerial guidelines, makes it difficult for the many parties involved to effectively manage their respective parts of the drug sector. Although the sector has performed well in terms of availability of drugs, many problems can be fully or partly explained by the lack of a policy and legal framework within which the sector can further develop. Uncertainty about policy and legislation may have a negative impact on investments, particularly from abroad.

Limited guidelines for the supply of pharmaceuticals have been provided in the 1994 National Health Plan and expressed as objectives and targets to be achieved. The Plan mentions the need for provision of essential drugs in PHC. It also notes the issue of the cost of drugs, estimating that pharmaceuticals cost $17 million (in public sector) or about 13.3 percent of the total health service costs in 1992, and forecasts that this will fall to 11.1 percent of health costs by the year 2000. The projections however are based on an assumption of real economic growth and the Plan falls short of providing solutions for issues effecting drugs costs.

The percentage is also incorrectly calculated since MOH drug expenditure is estimated at $61 million. The next Health Plan, now under early development, must address the issue of pharmaceutical supplies since they are not only costly but also necessary for the credibility of the health services.

The many pressing priorities in health and other sectors for both policy development and legislation may make it infeasible to press for early adoption of an NDP and a new legislation. However, an interim measure to start the process of drafting a national drug policy and drug legislation, and to begin consultations to this end, would have substantial benefits. It would provide sector leaders with some opinion on the direction in which policy and legislation should move, and will assure wider consultation in preparation for the time when prospects are good for a cabinet presentation.

THE DOMESTIC PHARMACEUTICAL INDUSTRY

There are seven drug companies in the West Bank; in Gaza Strip there is one small plant, and a medium–sized plant nearing completion. All companies are public share companies, although some are family based. In 1996, total value in ex–factory prices was estimated at $20 million. The largest company, Birzeit–Palestine Pharmaceutical, had 180 employees and reported a good profit on sales of about $9 million. Companies with less turnover are suffering from the small size of the market, competition for government contracts, and the loss of purchasing power. Exports to other countries are negligible.

While none of the factories have certificates of GMP, some are believed to be very close to qualifying and the Middle East Pharmaceutical Co. in Gaza Strip is being constructed to GMP standards. All factories formulate their products with imported raw materials and other ingredients. They all market their products as branded generics, with none producing brand–name drugs under license. Most of the factories have a large number of products.

Together, the eight factories produce 725 different branded generics, with Birzeit–Palestine leading with 221 products, followed by Jerusalem Pharmaceutical with 114. With only 12 branded generics, Al-Razi Chemical is the smallest. Many of the products are combination drugs, those that have two or more active ingredients. Of 502 drugs analyzed in 1995, 23 percent had two active ingredients and 24 percent had three or more. WHO does not recommend the use of combination products as they contribute little or nothing to drug therapy. They are marketed primarily for purposes of product differentiation in order to gain market share for the individual company and are more expensive than single–ingredient drugs. Steps should be taken to gradually remove combination products from the market, particularly those with no scientifically proven advantage.

Plant capacity utilization is low - Birzeit–Palestine Co. reports capacity utilization of only 35 percent. A number of factors combine to produce a non-competitive drug manufacturing sector. There are many producers compared to the size of the market, barriers to export are nearly complete, and there is a need for production of many small batches. In addition, Israeli registration requirements and the high-priced Israeli pharmaceutical industry effectively shields WBG drug producers from low-cost competition. As a result, production costs may be two to three times higher than those of foreign, low-cost generic manufacturers. A 15 percent allowance for domestic manufacturers will, in a few cases, be needed to award a contract to a local company.

Because production costs are high, the companies do not have good export prospects. When barriers to imports from non–Israeli companies are lifted, the drug manufacturing sector is thus likely to come under considerable pressure. In order to make the industry competitive in the branded-generic market, a number of changes will be necessary. Capacity utilization will have to increase considerably, batch sizes enlarged, and raw materials procurement consolidated to obtain better prices. The industry may also need to reduce the number of products manufactured at each plant. Factories will also need to qualify for and obtain the GMP certification.

The cost of introducing GMP is not negligible and may further diminish the industry's competitiveness. The MOH and the manufacturers association will likely decide to adopt GMP guidelines from the Arab Union of the Manufacturers of Pharmaceuticals and Medical Appliances. The Arab GMP requirements are higher and more costly than WHO requirements.

The local market, even with economic growth, is too small to sustain the present industry, not least in view of expansion plans.

When the social and political situation stabilizes, it would be useful for the industry to conduct a detailed feasibility study in order to asses means of increasing both its competitiveness and export orientation. MOH cannot indefinitely subsidize the industry through allowances and prices that are substantially higher in the private sector. With open borders, the industry is likely to face stiff competition from at least Egypt and Jordan and possibly from other countries with generic drug production.

NATIONAL LISTS OF ESSENTIAL DRUGS

There is as yet no official list of essential drugs. A committee has drafted a list which includes about 600 drugs, based on the principles of WHO's model lists, which has 250 drugs. Further consultations are needed prior to approval and publication of the draft list. Presently the exact number of drugs on the market is not known but according to UNICEF the figure was as high as 1,626 in 1993. However, pharmacy administration estimates that there may be as many as 4,000 drugs presently available.

Over the years there has been a trend towards the use of limited lists. MOH operates with about 600 different items and other agencies are even more restrictive. UNRWA follows WHO's model list very closely, with only about 250 drugs. UNRWA's experience with a limited list, standard treatment schedules, training and supervision has been positive in terms of availability, therapeutic results and patient satisfaction. At the primary health care (PHC) level this was achieved at a cost of about $1.20 per person in 1996, for the 1.678 million refugees covered by UNRWA services. Many NGO service providers also operate with limited lists. The Palestine Red Crescent Society (PRCS) used WHO's list prior to the peace process and now has a PHC list of only 67 drugs. Donors such as Pharmaciens sans Frontières and many others restrict their drug procurement to essential drugs.

The health sector appears to be ready for the introduction of a national list of essential drugs, which should be constructed by level of health care. The list for PHC could have 40-60 drugs and for secondary care 80-100 drugs; the full list should contain no more than 250-300 drugs and vaccines. Special provision must be made for drugs needed for rare conditions, and for patients who have started treatment abroad. A solution must also be found for the use of very expensive and sophisticated drugs for the relatively few patients who benefit from these.

The national list of essential drugs should be introduced and implemented gradually. Introduction, which should start in PHC centers, will require training and should be complemented by well-tested standard treatment protocols and careful monitoring. Consideration should also be given to introducing incentives for prescribers and dispensers. This could be in the form of training or promotion, or perhaps as a small share of savings from the drug budget. Implementation must be facilitated by public information and a thorough introduction of the principles and practice of the concept of essential drugs and the rational use of drugs. Because resistance to the essential drugs concept should be anticipated, measures to deal with it could be put in place prior to implementation. UNRWA's management of essential drugs in health centers has been a very cost effective approach to drug management with a limited list and should be disseminated and adapted to MOH clinics.

DRUG ADMINISTRATION

The pharmaceutical sector is regulated and administered by the General Administration of Pharmacy (GAP) in Gaza City and Ramallah. The Administration is headed by a Director General and Deputy Director General. The Deputy Director General reports, for practical reasons, to the Deputy Minister of Health. Prior to April 1994 the drug sector was almost completely under the control of the Israeli civil administration. Some functions, such as control of imports, are still under Israeli control.

Transfer of pharmaceutical control began in April, 1995 with the appointment of the Director General, who quickly started to develop the drug administration apparatus. This apparatus compromises eight divisions in Gaza and an office in Ramallah, with five divisions covering all areas of drug administration. GAP has now assumed most of the regulatory functions. Close contact is maintained between the two offices to coordinate rules and regulations.

Both GAP offices suffer from severe resource constraints. The skeleton staff administers everything from procurement, storage and distribution to inspection of factories and pharmacies, as well as registrations and quality control. There is no computer system linking the different functions and no drug information system for professionals or the public. There is a severe lack of senior technical staff, and present staff due to years of isolation, lack the professional experiences needed for development of a modern drug regulatory agency. Office space and storage capacity are lacking, and there are serious shortages of equipment, furniture and transport for the two central medical stores (CMSs). Funds for testing of special drugs like hormones, anticancer drugs and immunosuppressants are either absent or wholly inadequate.

The registration process has now been taken over completely. Drug applications are reviewed according to requirements and criteria defined by GAP. While all drugs which meet the criteria can in principle be registered, a committee may review an application to determine whether a drug is "needed" or if its price is reasonable. A negative determination by the committee on either of these issues is grounds for rejection of an application. Registration takes place in both Gaza and Ramallah. There are at present about 450 products registered in Gaza Strip and 750 in the West Bank, covering both public and private markets. Administration offices in Gaza and Ramallah share information and recognize drugs registered by the other office.

All drugs must be registered before they enter the WBG market. However, some Israeli companies are negligent in this respect. Other foreign companies register through their Palestinian agents. The registration fee is $300, with re–registration required after five years. Quality control is a part of the registration process. GAP presently uses the Center for Environmental and Occupational Health Laboratories at Birzeit University for all its drug testing, and anticipates establishing its own quality control facilities in the planned Public Health Laboratory. Drugs bought on tender or through MOH contracts are in principle tested before marketing, as are donated drugs. Major donors also arrange for testing of drugs procured abroad (UNRWA) or locally (Pharmaciens sans Frontières and many others).

Although the Birzeit University laboratory cannot fully test biological and hormonal substances or bioavailability, the quality of drugs in the market is believed to be acceptable. When a fully developed pharmacy administration is in place, including a quality control laboratory, increasing the reliance on GMP for ensuring quality may be advisable. GAP could then restrict testing to random samples, and to be used in case of doubt about a particular product's quality. To implement such a regime, a strong inspection system covering manufacturers, importers, drug stores and pharmacies would be needed.

The pharmacy administration and drug regulatory system clearly needs strengthening. A modest input may go a long way towards safeguarding the quality of pharmaceuticals in the market and could be a cheap insurance in a sector covering drugs worth over $50 million a year.

ESTIMATION OF PHARMACEUTICAL REQUIREMENTS

Estimations of public sector drug requirements are based on a combination of past consumption and availability of resources. The MOH allocates funds for drugs and consumables from its annual budget and allocated about $28 million in 1996. Quantities of drugs needed are estimated at 110 percent of past consumption for each health care facility; this automatic increase is intended to account for expanding population and services. There is therefore no linkage between morbidity patterns and service statistics (i.e., number of inpatients, outpatients, age distribution etc.) in determining drug requirements.

The past consumption method is widely used and has some merit, particularly in stable conditions of supply and demand. However, it also lends itself to distortions between medical needs and actual supply. Basing supplies on past consumption, all other things being equal, tends to reward the bigger consumers also. When only past consumption is used to determine supply, irrational prescribing may even be reinforced rather than controlled.

Requirements in the private sector are a composite of retail pharmacy projections of demand as well as the suppliers (drug stores, agents and manufacturers) estimation of the demand in the private market.

In order to match the real medical needs in the public sector with the supply of pharmaceuticals, it may soon be advisable to include morbidity patterns as part of the system of ascertaining drug requirements. This can be done on a pilot basis, using a few hospitals and clinics to test the degree to which such a system would improve drug therapy and/or save money. WHO has a tested methodology for estimating requirement and may be called upon for both testing, guidelines and equipment.

DRUG PRICING, COST OF DRUG CONSUMPTION AND FINANCING

The price of drugs for the public sector is in principle determined by competition. All qualified bidders have their offers examined by MOH's technical committee. The contract is awarded based on the best price, together with an assessment of the product and the manufacturer's past performance. If there are no bids for a product, three quotations are invited and a negotiated price is arrived at within a ceiling of NIS 25,000. MOH is reasonably successful in obtaining prices for many products around the international average for generic products but for some products it pays considerably higher prices (see Table A 12.2 for a comparison of MOH tender prices, UNRWA prices, retail pharmacy prices and international prices for the ten large volume products).

UNRWA obtains the lowest prices of all agencies in the WBG. Their prices for several products are very low, and in some cases even below international or UNICEF prices. NGOs often buy on tender and are assumed to obtain prices close to those of the Ministry. However, it may depend on their volume and ability to negotiate rebates etc. Their prices are outside the scope of this study.

Prices in the retail pharmacy sector in West Bank are determined by the Ministry of Health together with the Syndicate of Pharmacists. [77] Manufacturers, wholesalers and agents sell their products at the price they think the market will bear. Local prices are generally some 20-30 percent below Israeli prices and even lower than those of imported brand-name drugs.

The company prepares price lists indicating the price to the pharmacy and the patient and seeks MOH approval. The retail price is the ex-factory price plus 25 percent profit margin for the pharmacy and with 17 percent VAT (Value Added Tax) added. The factory or wholesaler post this price on each package and are not allowed to give rebates to the patients. Wholesalers have no specific mark up. They also charge for their service what the private pharmacy market will bear.

Pharmacy drug prices are considered high by the general public. They are indeed high when compared with international and MOH tender prices. Prices may increase, on similar products, by a factor of two or more. The price comparison in Table A 12.2 is not entirely fair to the retail sector, as the price calculations are based on units of 100s or 1,000s, whereas most retail pharmacies dispense drugs in packages with a course of treatment. However, prices are high compared to other countries at the same level of economic development and are in part influenced by the high retail prices prevailing in the Israeli market.

There is pressure on the MOH to increase price levels in the private sector. Two months ago, the pharmaceutical manufacturers attempted to increase overall prices by 20-25 percent. Price negotiations following these increases resulted in a lowering of the price increases to 10 percent. Such price increases require negotiations between several parties: The Manufacturers Association, Syndicate of Pharmacists, Ministry of Commerce, Ministry of Industry and of course the MOH. Such price increases may be justified on the grounds that the local industry must pay for their raw materials in foreign currencies.

Drug consumption in WBG is high compared to other countries at the same level of economic development. Consumption per capita is about 50 percent that of Israel, which has a much stronger economy and is about the same level as in Jordan, which has a somewhat stronger economy. However, drug consumption in Jordan is considered out of control and efforts are being made to reduce the cost of drugs in both the public and private sector. Egypt provides an interesting example. In 1996, drug consumption per capita was between US$14-15, and has steadily declined from a high of US$17 in 1987. As stated earlier, the fastest growing item of expenditure for MOH is the cost of drugs, vaccines, reagents and consumables. Such a high increase is not sustainable even in the near term, and certainly not in the medium- and long term.

---

[77] Prices in Gaza Strip are determined by a committee which consists of Ministries of Health, Commerce and Industry, etc. There are no Syndicates of Pharmacists in Gaza Strip.

Drugs are also a financial burden on households. In 1996 the Palestinian Central Bureau of Statistics, in its estimate of average monthly household expenditure on health, found that half of all expenditure goes on drugs and vitamins. A household will spend JD 10 each month, or JD 120 per year (US$168). With a household size of 6.9 persons, this means an average annual outlay of about US$24 per person. This is a very high figure posing considerable burden on the individual and his family, and would be even higher if refugees, who have access to free drugs, are excluded.

It is very difficult to determine the total value of drug consumption in the WBG. Budgets and expenditures for drugs are often combined with consumables and the drug costs cannot be desegregated. The volume of drugs imported to the private sector is not recorded by the administration, nor is it easy to determine the value of drugs supplied through the NGOs' health services. The following is the best estimate that the study could produce.

Table A 12.1: Estimate of Total Drug Consumption in West Bank and Gaza

Subsector	Total consumption (US$ million)	Percent of total
Ministry of Health	17.5	37
UNRWA	2	4
Nongovernmental Organizations	8	17
Private Sector	20	42
Total	47	100

Source: Ministry of Health, World Bank Staff Estimates.

The two first amounts are well documented, however there is uncertainty regarding estimates for the NGO and private sector. There are about 250 NGO facilities, but many do not provide drugs. Some of the larger NGOs', provide large amounts such as Pharmaciens sans Frontières about US$1 million; PRCS, about US$800,000 (include disposables); and MAP around US$1 million. Small NGOs provide anything from US$100.000 to much less. According to informed people, these estimates seem to be of the right magnitude.

The estimate for the private sector is the subject of more dispute. Estimates by the administration place private sales at US$20 million, while UNICEF's report of 1993 suggested a total retail price of US$55 million. Pharmacists and drug stores report that sales have fallen in the last year or two, but hardly to a level of US$20 million. Household expenditure on drugs of $24 per person seems to confirm a much higher level of private sector expenditure, since a large part of the population is receiving drugs free or at very low cost. US$24 per person per year would indicate a private sector expenditure of the similar magnitude as UNICEF's estimate i.e. US$55 million. Deducting MOH and UNRWA drug costs and taking into account the drug fees in the NGO and MOH services and a reduction in purchasing power of about 10 percent, would give a figure of perhaps US$40 million. Using these rough estimates the annual drug bill could be as much as US$ 67 million. This would mean an annual per capita consumption of drugs of US$29.

Efforts and interventions to reduce the total drug bill in WBG must be made a priority for short term. The inefficiencies in the system, from registration, pricing, procurement, storage, distribution, prescription and use, provide a wide range of opportunities for cost containment (for possible savings see Table A 12.3).

MOH's drug and medical consumables budget is financed from general revenue sources and is in 1997 expected to reach 32.5 percent of total MOH expenditure. There is some co-payment by patients. Patients with health insurance obtain their in-patient drugs completely free of charge. OPD drugs are paid for with a flat fee of NIS 3 per drug item or unit (a unit corresponds to a normal course of treatment). Drugs for children under three years cost only NIS 1. In the case of a few expensive drugs the patient may be required to pay up to 50 percent of the cost price. Clinics have a petty cash of NIS 500 to use for local purchase in case of stock-shortages. There may be some unfairness in the application of a flat fee for very low cost drugs. Many essential drugs cost much less than NIS 3 for a treatment course, and with the flat fee the patient is in a way being taxed or is indirectly subsidizing the more expensive drugs. Many countries link co-payment fully or partly to the cost of the drug. It may, at some point in the future, be advisable to review the present co-payment scheme and perhaps find a fairer system.

UNRWA provides all drugs free of charge and will refund part of the cost of drugs procured in private pharmacies or used in in-patient care, for those drugs not available in UNRWA's own stores. Many NGOs charge the actual cost of drugs to patients who can pay, but will allow non-insured or poor patients to obtain drugs for part-payment or free of charge.

The private pharmacies charge a fixed price. There is little discounting, and free drugs cannot be obtained through the retail pharmacies. Some pharmacies report that poor patients sometimes leaves without a drug due to high price.

All co-payments for drugs are collected at the dispensary and the revenue, lumped together with other payments, go through MOH's directorate of finance to the Ministry of Finance. The accounts do not show the magnitude of co-payments for drugs. In addition to the fees collected at MOH facilities, the MOF receive considerable revenue from the 17 percent VAT added to the pharmacy price.

DRUG PROCUREMENT

The MOH buys 85 percent of its drug needs through two annual tenders. The remaining 15 percent is bought directly following requests for quotations. Direct purchasing is used when there are no bidders for the required items. The largest direct purchase is for immunosuppressants at about $2 million annually.

The Ministry advertises its tender in the local newspapers. Eligible companies and agents then buy the tender documents from the Ministry. Bids are examined by a technical committee which advises the tender committee on quality and reputation of suppliers. Price is the determining factor in awarding a contract. In the first tender in 1997, 50 percent was awarded to the lowest bidder and 30 percent was awarded to companies which were the only bidders. Other considerations are delivery terms, reputation of the company and past experience with the product. In most cases the second or third lowest bidder will then get the contract.

In view of the constraints imposed by Israeli registration requirements for imported drugs, the MOH does quite well in terms of prices. Table A 12.2 shows that, of 10 high volume drugs, the Ministry in two cases obtained prices below international indicator prices for generics and in most other cases was only marginally above. This is quite impressive when seen that the MOH price also includes delivery to the warehouse. There are, however, instances where the

Ministry buys at very high prices. It may be advisable for MOH to regularly compare international indicator prices with those they obtain to ensure that they are operating in the right price range.

The 15 percent allowance for local manufacturers is rarely used. In the last tender only six items out of 116 required this subsidy in order that the contract could be awarded to a local manufacturer. This is fortunate, since it is not MOH's role to subsidize industry.

UNRWA uses international competitive bidding and consolidates all its drug requirements for Palestinian refugees (Syria, Jordan, Egypt and WBG) in one large tender. They obtain exceptionally good prices, as shown in Table A 12.2.

Table A 12.2: Prices of Selected Drugs in West Bank and Gaza and International Prices (1996)

Organization			Ministry of Health	UNRWA	Pharmacy	International Price
Drug	Strength	Unit	NIS ($)	US ($)	NIS ($)	US $
Amoxycillin	500 mg	1,000	210 (61.8)		750 (220)	60.00
Acetylsalisylic Acid	100 mg	1,000	133 (39)		275 (81)	3.00
Acetylsalisylic Acid	300 mg	1,000		5.5 (500 mg)		3.60
Ampicillin Injection	1 g	Vial	1.64 (0.48)	0.279	8.4 (2.5)	0.37
Cephalexin	500 mg	1,000	327 (96)	120	1,375 (404)	132.00
Carbamazepine	200 mg	1,000	170 (50)			30.00
Diazepam	5 mg	1,000	26 (7.6)		175 (51)	3.00
Diazepam Injection	5 mg/ml	2 ml vial	1.17 (0.38)	0.064	2.6(0.76)	0.09
ORS	1 Sachet		1.24 (0.36)	0.08	6.13 (1.80)	0.10
Dextrose 5 Percent	5%	500 ml	3.99 (1.2)			1.35
Ferreous Salt + Folic Acid	60 mg + 0.26	1,000	94 (27.61)			3.50
Glibenclamide	5 mg	1,000	24 (7.1)		624 (183.5)	5.00
Insulin (Human insulin)	100 IU/ml	10 ml	28 (8.2)	(BI) 4.8; (HI) 8.1		(BI) 5.90
Mebentazole	100 mg	1,000	180 (53)		1760 (517)	6.00
Metronidazole	500 mg	Vial	5.51 (1.62)		21.5 (6.3)	1.10
Nefidipine	10 mg	1,000	130 (38.2)		326 (96)	22.80
Oxytocin Inj.	10 IU	Vial	2.85 (0.84)			0.13

Note: BI = Beef Insulin; HI = Human Insulin. VAT (Value Added Tax) = 17 %.
Source: Ministry of Health, UNRWA, World Bank Staff Estimates, Management Sciences for Health.

DRUG DISTRIBUTION

Drugs are stored and distributed through numerous channels. MOH operates two central warehouses. The Ramallah CMS is located in a two-storied, former cement store (1,800 square meters), and has very little equipment and transportation. The Gaza store is smaller and is housed on the compound of the Shifa hospital, but also with very little store equipment and is difficult to access. There are satellite stores for equipment and disposables. In Gaza a new, large store is under construction. The 1,300 square meters ground floor is nearing completion, but funds are lacking for its completion and for the building of the first floor for equipment and offices. Both stores are very well stocked, nearly to choking point. The Ramallah CMS, for instance, in mid-May had an inventory holding of about US$6 million - sufficient for six months or more. Computer systems and modern store management systems are sorely lacking.

MOH drugs, vaccines, disposables and reagents are distributed to hospitals and district stores on a bimonthly basis, based on requests from facilities. These request sheets contain information on stocks of each item and the request for replenishment. The CMS will then evaluate the request based on past performance and availability of the specific item. This often results in a severe reduction in the amount actually delivered. The requesting health facility is not guided by a budget, but has some information on the quantities of drugs and consumables, which they can expect to receive during the year. Hospital and clinical pharmacies keep stocks and distribute these regularly (daily) to wards and OPD clinics. However, the district central store delivers drugs to its satellite clinics monthly.

UNRWA operates two major stores. They receive their drugs and consumables directly from UNRWA's international procurement program and rarely supplement with local procurement due to its higher cost. UNRWA's stores are computerized and follow modern drug store management systems. They distribute on a regular basis to all their clinics based on actual needs.

The UNRWA drug management system is a good model of how an effective supply organization can work, even under difficult circumstances. The UNRWA drug system should be adapted for MOH use and their experience transferred through training or perhaps exchange of staff. As it is now, there is virtually no collaboration between the UNRWA and the MOH system.

Many NGOs operate their own stores and distribute either to their own clinics or, in the case of foreign agents, to the clinics which come under their program. Most procure locally, in spite of the price. The barrier to low-cost procurement is the difficulty with regards to registration and import via Israel.

The local pharmaceutical manufacturers supply directly to retail pharmacies, often on long-term credit. Imported drugs are distributed from the approximately 50 drug wholesalers and distributors. Most of these have small stores where they stock the drugs they anticipate will be needed in the retail pharmacy store. Some are agents for big pharmaceutical houses in Europe or act as sub-agents for Israeli companies. Some act only as middlemen for MOH contracts, submitting the bid on behalf of the companies they represent. However, they do not provide a service in the form of warehouses and distribution.

The storage and distribution systems have contributed to the safety of supplies and the good and regular availability of drugs in most facilities. Indeed, the stock levels are very high both in the public and private sector, whereas UNRWA operates a leaner system. The supply system, however, does not always assure that the peripheral clinics have a good stock of drugs. A consequence of this is that patients then need to return to the doctor to get the prescription changed or get a referral slip to the district pharmacy or a private pharmacy. One reason for non-availability, however, is that some doctors prescribe drugs which are not on the MOH clinical drugs list.

There is merit, in times of conflict and border closures, in maintaining a high inventory level. However, this is always at a cost in terms of tied-up capital and not least in the risk of having many drugs expire before use. In view of the relatively small territory of WBG and the size of the population, one can question the need for such a large number of stores and distributors. There may be some merit in trying to be restrictive in the granting of licenses for agents and perhaps also in attempts to encourage organizations to combine their procurement, storage and distribution systems.

DRUG PRESCRIPTION, DISPENSING AND CONSUMPTION

This component of drug use represents a multitude of problems and real opportunities for improvements and savings.

The 1993 UNICEF study on the supply of pharmaceuticals clearly demonstrated problems in the prescription and use of drugs. It recorded excessive use of antibiotics and the use of many inappropriate combination drugs, as well as overuse of vitamins and mineral preparations. Overprescription and overuse of drugs is widespread throughout the world, and the Middle East has more than its share of this problem. This study recorded that in 1991 an estimated 25 million packages of drugs were prescribed to the population, corresponding to about 12 courses of treatment per capita per year.

Prescribing practices have recently been examined by the pharmacy administration (Jan-March 1997) in six MOH institutions (hospitals and urban clinics). The reports have recorded numerous problems. There is widespread over-prescription of drugs - the result of a vicious circle where patients expect or demand drugs from the doctors and the doctors know that patients expect them to prescribe. Indeed, it is widely believed that a doctor's status among his patients is partly determined by his ability or willingness to prescribe powerful drugs. There is also strong demand for injections and suppositories, not least in the private clinics. These are much more expensive than tablets or capsules, which nearly always have the same therapeutic effect.

Many doctors prescribe several drugs or combination drugs, where one ingredient would often have been sufficient. This may be a reflection of the short time spent in examination of the patient. Antibiotics, combination drugs or other inappropriate combinations then act as substitute for a good diagnosis and dialogue with the patient. Several studies have shown that up to 50 percent of PHC patients are not really in need of medication. Yet, few leave without one.

One problem is also the doctors' preference for brand-name prescriptions or products from a specific producer. In the above MOH study, it was found that the number of drugs per prescription ranged from 1.8 to 3.1 and that nearly all were brand names. One hospitals had no single generic prescription and the highest percentage was only 8 percent. This is of lesser importance in MOH clinics, since the Ministry buys by generic name. However, the reliance on brand names produces patient loyalty to a specific product, even when he or she moves to another clinic or seeks treatment in the private sector.

Doctors in private practice are very particular about using brand-name drugs for their patients. Some even insist that the patient return to their clinic to show that he/she actually received the prescribed drug. This contributes to higher costs to both the patient and society, since generic substitution is not allowed under pharmacy law. In the case of patients who cannot afford an expensive brand product, the pharmacist or the patient must contact the doctor to get his permission to dispense a lower-cost branded-generic or generic product. The pharmacist, of course, also has an incentive for dispensing the highest priced drugs, since he gets 25 percent on top of the purchase price. Although it takes about the same amount of work to dispense a package of low-cost generics than an expensive brand-name drug, the pharmacist is rewarded for the latter rather than for the former.

There is pressure on the doctors and perhaps also on the pharmacists to function at the expensive end of the drug spectrum. The industry as well as the major importers use medical representatives for information on their products. The sales promotion may take the form of many samples, which can be passed on to patients, or loyalty to a product or company may be developed through seminars, travels and other means. There are WHO guidelines for the ethical promotion of pharmaceuticals. It could be well worth the effort to consider these in the drafting of a national drug policy or drug legislation. Education and licensing of medical representatives may also safeguard against unethical marketing.

The above study and other reports also point to a widespread belief among the population that there is a drug for (nearly) all ills. The high priority assigned to drugs is clearly demonstrated in the statistics regarding monthly household expenditure. Drugs and vitamins account for by far the largest cost, at about 50 percent of total cost or US$160 per year. This is followed by the cost of physician services at US$70 per household each year. The physician's visit is, in many cases, for the purpose of obtaining a prescription. The study shows there is also widespread belief that injections and suppositories are better than tablets and capsules. In addition many patients believe that imported medicines are "better" than locally manufactured products.

RETAIL PHARMACIES

There are a total of 560 retail pharmacies: 358 in West Bank and 202 in Gaza Strip. This gives a ratio of retail pharmacies to population of 1:4.071. Registered pharmacists in West Bank and in Gaza Strip can apply for a license and if the pharmacist meets the requirements of the pharmacy laws applicable in his/her geographical location, he or she will be granted a license provided the premises are 32 square meters or bigger. Until recently it was a requirement in West Bank that a new pharmacy must be situated at least 40 meters away form an established pharmacy. In Gaza Strip the required distance was 200 meters. A compromise has now been reached and MOH has decreed that the distance should be no less than 100 meters between pharmacies.

The ratio of pharmacies to population is high compared to European countries with greater population density (Denmark 1: 15.000, Norway: 1:13,000), but not to, for instance, a neighboring country like Jordan with a ratio of 1: 3,451 or Egypt with 1: 4,400. However, the retail pharmacy sector is under considerable strain. Quite a few pharmacies in Gaza Strip have been forced to close, but this has not prevented other pharmacists from opening up.

There are too few patients in need of private pharmacy products who are able to pay. The market is very small since most patients get medicines free (UNRWA and some NGOs) or, in public sector facilities for a small flat fee. The last few years' decline in the economy has also been severely felt in the private pharmacy sector. Many pharmacies have only 10 to 20 clients per day and even bigger ones may not have more than 30-40. A few well-located pharmacies may, however, have hundreds of clients daily. Many patients shop around for discounts or return empty-handed when they realize the cost of the medicine. Pharmacy owners may be tempted to dispense drugs without a prescription, although the degree to which such practice is used is not known.

With few other employment opportunities, pharmacists will be tempted to open a pharmacy to make sure that they obtain a license. They may be investing in the long-term prospects, in the hope that patients and customers for perfumes and other toiletries will give them some turnover and perhaps even some profit. There are no legal tools for the Ministry to reduce the number of pharmacies. The old but still valid pharmacy laws give those who comply with the requirements the right to receive a license and operate a private pharmacy.

The proliferation of pharmacies, however, have not improved the drug retail service. The few times a year (or month) when a family needs drugs does not require the presence of a pharmacy every one hundred meters. It is also wasteful in terms of having well-educated pharmacists severely underemployed in their profession, as well as in terms of tying up capital which could be put to more productive use. The basic problem seems to be that there are too many pharmacy graduates for society's needs. The WBG area has a total of 1,240 registered pharmacists (ratio of pharmacists to pop. 52:100,000).

There are no easy solutions to this problem. It may be tempting to allow the market forces to determine who will survive. Some other, albeit richer, countries in the region allow the virtual free establishment of pharmacies. However, most countries have a rationing system which takes into account population density and related factors. Too many pharmacies may lead to undesirable malpractice in the form of dispensing drugs without prescription, pushing higher-price drugs or, as is the case in some countries, buying smuggled drugs and combining their sales with tax evasion. The cost of inefficiency in having more pharmacies than needed will, one way or another, have to be passed on to patients in the form of higher prices or unnecessary consumption.

It would seem necessary to relieve the pressure on the pharmacy owners through MOH intervention. A first, though rather long-term, solution would be to reduce the annual intake to the pharmacy schools, which is presently at 80 in each of the two existing schools. Consequently, this may lead to the closure of either the West Bank or Gaza school. If implemented for a sustained period, this may bring the ratio of pharmacists to population closer to what is needed and financially viable. A somewhat shorter-term solution, at least for new pharmacies, would be to tighten the rules on the size of premises and the years of practice required before a pharmacist can apply for a license. A new regulation may also require the presence of the pharmacy owner for at least part of the working day and require that only registered pharmacists are hired for dispensing of medicines. The use of non-pharmacy staff for dispensing should be completely disallowed.

COST CONTAINMENT IN THE DRUG SECTOR

There are many opportunities for savings in the supply and use of drugs. Some can be implemented with relative ease and may still contribute to cost containment. Other measures are more difficult to formulate and implement. The biggest savings require both time, commitment and some luck to achieve. When cost containment measures are put in place, there are always groups or individuals who resist or feel hurt, not least if they are seeing their profits reduced. However, much resistance can be countered, while keeping in mind that the patients should continue to get the best possible treatment.

Many countries have gone through a partial or comprehensive drug sector reform. The results have in many cases been very encouraging, whether in developed or developing countries. The experiences have demonstrated the potential for savings and some of these are listed below. The percentages indicate the maximum achievable and therefore do not necessarily add up. Each saving has consequences for the savings in other elements, and the percentages merely indicate what could be achieved if a specific intervention was carried out in isolation. The total savings could well be in the range of 30 - 40 percent.

Table A 12.3 : Potential Savings in Drug Sector Reform

Activity	Saving (percent)
Implement National Drug Policy and Legislation	5
Introduce Essential Drug List at All Health Care Levels	5 - 10
Improve MOH Procurement	10
Implement Standard Treatment Protocols in Public Health Facilities	5 - 10
Introduce and Enforce Generic Substitution	5 - 10
Improve Storage and Distribution Management	5 - 10
Shift from Injections to Tablets and Capsules When Justified	2 - 5
Remove Inappropriate Drugs from the Market	3 - 5
Total Rationalization Of Drug Sector	**30 - 40**

RECOMMENDATIONS

Recommendations following the study of the pharmaceutical sector are grouped in three categories, not necessarily in order of priority or importance. Rather, an attempt has been made to categorize the recommendations as those which can be implemented soon and with relative ease (Category I); those which will require more time and preparation and may be more difficult to implement (Category II); and finally the long-term activities (Category III), necessary to improving the performance of the sector but which may be difficult to implement, or which may require the involvement of many sectors and interest groups:

In Category I

- Early approval and implementation of the essential drugs list, starting in primary health care of the public sector;

- Finalization and introduction of standard treatment protocols at all levels of care;

- Steps are taken to have the Israeli requirements on registration of imported drugs lifted for products from GMP certified manufacturers being supplied to the MOH;

- Introduction of stricter requirements for the establishment of private pharmacies;

- Intake to pharmacy schools is severely restricted and the closure of one pharmacy school is considered;

- Plans for computerization of central drug stores' management are implemented;

- Improved methods for estimation of drug requirements are introduced;

- Process is begun whereby combination drugs (drugs containing two, three or more active ingredients) are removed from the market as they become due for re-registration.

It is further recommended, once the category I recommendations are under implementation that:

In Category II

- Essential drugs lists for secondary public health facilities is implemented and also introduced into NGO primary care services;

- Capacity of the pharmaceutical sector administration is strengthened though additional technical staff and managerial training;

- Ramallah Central Medical Store is renovated and equipped and first floor of Gaza Store is completed and equipped;

- Proper Quality Control Laboratory is established;

- GMP certifications are established;

- System of co-payments for drugs is reviewed and streamlined;

- Drug pricing and fixed pricing for pharmacies is reviewed and streamlined.

For longer-term results, it is recommended that:

In Category III

- Essential drugs lists are implemented in the tertiary health care as well as in NGO hospitals;

- Scheme for generic substitution is developed, tested and implemented;

- National Drug Plan is drafted, discussed and approved by the legislative council;

- Modern drug legislation is drafted, approved and implemented;

- Regulations and guidelines for all elements of the pharmaceutical sector are drafted, discussed and implemented.

Table A 12.4: Cost Estimates for Pharmaceutical Sector Reform (US$ thousand)

Activity	Year		
	1	2	3
1. Implement National Drug Policy and Legislation			
Workshops	30	30	20
Technical Assistance	20	20	-
Printing, Distribution and Promotion	15	10	-
2. Introduce Essential Drug Lists at All Levels of Care			
Workshops	100	50	50
Technical Assistance	20	-	-
Printing, Distribution and Promotion	30	30	20
Study Tours	20	20	-
3. Improve Ministry of Health Procurement			
Training Abroad	30	30	-
Computer Equipment	10	-	-
4. Implement Standard Treatment Protocols In Public Health Facilities			
Workshops	50	30	10
Technical Assistance	30	-	-
Printing, Distribution and Promotion	30	15	10
5. Introduce And Enforce Generic Substitution			
Workshops	50	30	-
Technical Assistance	20	-	-
Printing, Distribution and Promotion	30	30	30
6. Improve Storage and Distribution Management			
Training Abroad	50	25	-
Computerization	30	20	10
Civil Works/Rehabilitation	200	50	50
7. Change in Clinical Practice (from injections to tablets etc.)			
Workshops	30	20	10
Technical Assistance	15	-	-
Printing, Distribution and Promotion	20	15	10
8 Remove Inappropriate Drugs from the Market			
Technical Assistance	15	10	10
Printing, Distribution, Promotion and Monitoring	15	10	10

Source: World Bank Staff Estimates.

Appendix 13: DEVELOPMENT OF A LEGISLATIVE FRAMEWORK FOR HEALTH INSURANCE

INTRODUCTION

The establishment of a comprehensive health insurance system is stated as a goal in the National Health Plan for the Palestinian people (1994). Until now this goal has been only partly realized, and much work remains to establish adequate regulations in place[78]. A few options for and elements of a possible regulatory framework for a national health insurance system are described below. These will hopefully serve as a guide for future efforts by the Palestinian Authority (PA) to establish a national health insurance system.

OBJECTIVES OF A HEALTH INSURANCE SYSTEM

To finance and regulate health services, countries can opt either for a national health service paid by general revenues, or an insurance system paid by contributions of the insured. Experiences in Western European countries have shown that both ways can be effective in providing access to good quality care for the population for roughly comparable costs.[79] Health insurance has the advantage of clearly earmarking the funds allocated for health care, thereby making their transactions transparent to the population (the contributors know what they are paying, and for what services). In principle, health insurance funds are also less likely to be subject to *ad hoc* policy changes by political process (e.g., budget alterations), in contrast to national health services that are financed directly through government budgets.

Under the social insurance system, providers are more likely to be private or independent parastatal entities, unlike the national health services in which the providers usually come under the direct management of the government agency. However in most countries with social insurance programs, governments impose strict regulations for setting contribution rates as part of a general social and employment policies, and for the same reason restrict the basket of services reimbursed through social insurance. At the same time, systems with government-managed providers have been experimenting with a greater separation of provider and payers through the introduction of contractual relations and greater managerial autonomy for the public providers. As a result, the distinction between social insurance and national health services is becoming increasingly blurred.

Under whatever choice of health system, it is important to define the objectives and establish the legislative and regulatory framework of the health financing system. In the National Health Plan, the national health insurance program is described as: "an indemnity coverage against financial losses associated with the treatment of a health problem." [80] This statement focuses only on the financing aspects of the system, and does not capture the full scope

---

[78] For a brief description of the present state of health insurance, see, Piva, P., M.A. Hashish, and R. Zanoun, "The Palestinian Universal Social Health Insurance", West Bank and Gaza Strip, 1997.

[79] This is subject to some controversy: at least one study (J.P. Poullier, "Administrative Costs in Selected Industrial Countries." Health Care Financing Review (summer), 1992: 167-72) suggests that the administrative costs of managing a social insurance system might be higher than the costs associated with the management of general tax-based national health services.

[80] National Health Plan, 1994, Annex 2, p. ix.

of the objectives of a national insurance program. A more appropriate definition that is more in line with the health policy of the National Health Plan would be to describe the health insurance and its regulations as a means for guaranteeing access for the whole population to efficiently provided essential care (i.e. care for which there is an objective medical need and which is of proven effectiveness in relation to need). The mandate of the health insurance program could be further expanded to encompass a more pro-active role in reducing the avoidable health risks among the insured population: for example, through contracts with the providers, health insurance programs could actively promote an early detection of potential health threats and consequently provide preventive care or early treatment of disease.

Given the present economic situation in West Bank and Gaza (WBG), the Palestinian will first need to attend to cost-containment measures and other measures needed to improve the efficiency of the present delivery system before attempting major reforms into the organization of the health financing structure. An important first step in that process will be to estimate the real costs for the various services to be implemented in the future package of benefits of the insurance system. These data will form the basis for calculating the appropriate prices for contracting individual providers and estimating the contribution rates from the insurance beneficiaries. Subsidization of the insurance system from general revenues will likely continue to be an important means for ensuring a redistribution of resources across different categories of population: this is a common feature of most social insurance systems around the world.

CONTENTS OF THE HEALTH INSURANCE LEGISLATION

The following sections describe the key issues and topics that should be included in a health insurance legislation.

Legal Status of Health Insurance

The responsibilities of the PA, the Legislative Council and the Ministry of Health (MOH) must first be clearly articulated in relation to the health insurance system. One of the first question that must be settled in the health insurance legislation is the identification of the institution that will function as the health insurance agency: whether it should remain as a department or a division under the direct authority of the Ministry, or to be established as a separate agency outside of the Ministry.

If the agency is to be established outside the Ministry, then the relations between the MOH and the health insurance agency must be specified in terms of their respective managerial and oversight responsibilities and capacities. In doing so, particular attention must be given to role of the MOH in its oversight and regulatory capacity with respect to the health insurance agency, for example, through the review of the agency's management decisions, the evaluation of its financial performance, and the exercise of sanctions against any undesirable decision-making by the agency. The legislation should specify the reporting requirements of the health insurance agency in terms of the timing and levels and types of decisions must be submitted to the MOH for approval.

Alternatively, health insurance could be administered separately through a self-governing body (such as a mutual or sickness fund) under the oversight of a publicly regulated board comprising representatives drawn from various interest groups. As with the health insurance agency, the rights and responsibilities of the organization must clearly be defined, along with the oversight and regulatory functions for the MOH. The possibility of an appeal to a court or arbitration procedure must also be included in the formulation of the legal framework for these independent agencies or bodies (see below).

In defining the legal status of the health insurance agency or body, the broader legal framework must be taken into consideration. For example, the health insurance legislation should be consistent with the rules and regulations governing financial institutions, e.g., with respect to accounting and audit requirements of the insurance fund. In addition, the legislation should also be consistent with the specific laws pertaining to the licensing of health providers, investments in health facilities, quality assurance, importation of pharmaceuticals, and others. Some aspects of these laws could be incorporated into the health insurance legislation if they are closely related.

Given the small size of the Palestinian population, there seems to be little justification in having more than one agency in place. The agency could place several regional offices but managed under the jurisdiction of the central agency. Two separate agencies could be established respectively for the West Bank and Gaza Strip, but if this split is introduced then mechanisms should be put in place to redistribute resources between the two agencies to ensure that funding and provision of services between the two territories are equitable.

Coverage

The health insurance legislation should include provisions on the eligibility and coverage of the health insurance system. Some examples of how these eligibility criteria can be defined are presented below:

- all Palestinians, living in and outside the territories, defined by characteristics recognizable to the health insurance agency. Including Palestinians living outside the territories could cause administrative problems in collecting contributions and in dealing with the costs for services.
- only the residents of the territories
- residents temporarily staying outside (e.g., on holiday or business; civil servants of PA working temporarily outside the territories.)
- specific categories of the population to be automatically covered (e.g., the unemployed, workers earning below a minimum wage, social welfare recipients), or excluded (e.g., military personnel and their dependents).

Contributions

This section of the legislation describes the respective duties and responsibilities of the health insurance agency and the beneficiaries in terms of the beneficiary contributions to the insurance plan. The following list provides examples of items which could be included in this section:

Party responsible for paying the premiums:

- all covered insured persons
- only the heads of families (including a legal definition of the family unit)

- specialized agencies, such as Ministry of Social Welfare, pension funds

Means for collecting premiums:

- direct payments by individuals
- payroll deductions, or payments through employers
- payments through other agencies, such as social security agency, cooperatives, associations

Party responsible for determining contribution rates:

- the PA
- the MOH
- the health insurance agency
- patient/community representative

Methods for establishing contribution rates:

- income-dependent, up to a certain maximum
- income-independent or fixed rate
- as a combination of these two

Special categories of contributors.   The MOH or the health insurance agency could be delegated the authority to define a lower percentage or a lower fixed rate contribution for certain categories of the insured population, e.g., people over 65, students, people on a social welfare. These categories must be well-defined and easily recognizable in order to avoid administrative problems. However, since the determination of these special categories depend on social and political notion of fairness and justice, these will probably need to be ratified through some process.

Establishment of a common fund into which all contributions flow.   At   present,   all contributions from the government health insurance premiums are submitted directly to the Treasury. If a health insurance agency is established, it will be necessary to set up a separate fund into which all contributions are channeled, including contributions from the general taxation. As noted earlier, subsidies from general tax revenues will likely be a necessary feature of the health insurance fund as long as it remains under the government jurisdiction. An alternative to direct transfers from general revenues would be for the government or the MOH to act as guarantors for loans from commercial banks.

Payments

This section describes the expenditure items which the health insurance agency is allowed to make payments. Examples include:

- the administrative costs of the insurance fund
- the costs of health services covered in the benefits package
- payments for activities related to health service and health insurance pre-approved by the governing board or the PA/MOH, e.g., research on evaluation of health services, health education, community outreach programs, and preventive care programs.
- interests on loans

Benefits Package

This section describes the benefits package, or the services, to which the beneficiaries are entitled.

Designing the benefits package. The benefits package presently used by the PA/MOH is typical of a more global list of services that defines benefits in broad categories of service types, e.g., ambulatory care visits or hospitalization. These general descriptions do not provide sufficiently clear specification of the types of care the beneficiaries. They creates confusion on the part of the beneficiaries and leave few options on the part of the health-insurance agency to control costs and guarantee quality of services.

A more refined benefits package could be developed that specifies the services and types of care through the use of well-defined positive or negative lists. A positive list must specify precisely the kinds of services and pharmaceuticals to which the insured are entitled. For example, the patient does not have entitlement to drugs that are not included in the positive list. A negative list is often used in conjunction with a global description of services, e.g., the benefits could include all forms of hospitalization *excluding* cosmetic surgery or certain types of organ transplantation.

Determining the service providers. The definition of benefits must also include the description of providers and programs which are included in the list. For example, currently the government health insurance does not cover visits to private physicians. Some examples of the description of eligible service providers are given below:

- all available providers within the WBG, or all public providers and private providers with a written contract with the health insurance agency;
- overseas providers with contracts with the health insurance agency;
- the place where the service can be obtained, at home or in an institution, must also be specified (e.g., for mental health services, community based and institutional care are both currently covered by the government health insurance).

Specification of the providers depends on the types of contractual relations with the providers and provider payment systems in place. The legislation should allow sufficient flexibility to accommodate the changes in the system as the relationship between the health insurance agency and providers evolves.

Some health insurance systems require their beneficiaries to register with a specific primary health care clinic or a family doctor. By appointing a particular primary care giver as the gatekeeper for the insurance beneficiaries, it allows the insurance agency to follow more easily the utilization pattern of the provider (referrals, drug prescriptions, diagnostic tests) and control the moral hazard problems created by patients "shopping" around. This measure must be balanced by the need to protect the patients' right to choose their primary care giver.

Conditions for obtaining a special type of service. Some services could be provided under special conditions, e.g., overseas referrals for cases requiring treatment not available within WBG. The process by which these cases are approved should be specified, e.g.:

- proof of objective medical need
- written referral from qualified specialists
- approval of the health insurance agency before rendering the services
- cost sharing by the patient

Copayment system.   Different options exist for designing the copayment system.   They include: (i) a fixed amount per service, (ii) a percentage of the costs per service, (iii) all the costs over a certain amount paid for by the health insurance agency (limited reimbursement-system), or (iv) a combination of these. A copayment can be made income-dependent and a maximum amount of copayment per service (or for all services) per year can be formulated.

A general deductible system fits better in a reimbursement system (see below) since this form of payment is generally used by private insurers.

Payment of Benefits.   The benefits can be provided to the patients in two broadly different ways:

- <u>Reimbursement system</u>: In this system, the costs of services are first paid by the insured, and reimbursed by the insurance agency to the patient retrospectively upon submission of the bills. Such a system is usually used by private health insurers but it is costly to run since the insurer must review and reimburse individual bills.

- <u>Benefits in kind</u>:   In this system the beneficiary is entitled to services and does not have to make payments to the provider (except for copayments or deductibles). In such a system, the insurer deals directly with the provider (e.g. through contracts).   This system is administratively more efficient and it allows the insurers to keep track of the behavior of the providers.

Parties responsible for defining the benefits package.   In defining a package of benefits, the legislation should address the question of who decides about the content of the package and how often revisions should be made. These decisions should be made by multidisciplinary group with representatives from interested parties as well as representatives of key technical disciplines.

In situations of rapid changes, e.g., rapid progress in medical technology, reforms in the payment systems, changes in economic conditions, it is especially important to have in place a procedure that allows the benefits package to be revised quickly.   The system of negative lists in particular requires a rapid adjustment procedure.

The decisions on benefits package will involve a continual review of new technologies (including the review of cost effectiveness and cost benefits at individual and social levels). There should be in place a system for monitoring the existing services and technologies. Any use of technologies that are obsolete or not effective should be removed from the positive list of services or added to the negative list. Immediate savings can thus be achieved.

Contracts

Contracting services will likely become an increasingly important feature of the health insurance agency.   The legislation should be written in a way that encourages the health insurance agency to organize contracts efficiently and in sufficient number ensure good services for the beneficiaries. In the future, the public providers might also enter into contractual relations with the MOH or health insurance agency.

Some examples of the conditions which can be specified in a contract are listed below:

- the type of service to be delivered
- the way in which the service is given: only on strict indication and in the most efficient way, using as much as possible the accepted standards, protocols and clinical guidelines
- access to the provider: opening hours, on call during weekends etc., referring to a colleague when on holiday etc.
- the obligation to have a sufficient administration (concerning financial as well as patients records)
- the conditions under which the health insurance agency has access to the administration (as for example the medical advisor to the medical records when there are doubts about the "production-pattern" of the provider
- the billing process
- the timely and properly payment of the provider
- the information about the insured registered to the practice of the provider
- specification of the arbitration process

Separate attention must be paid to the tariffs (medical price) and the adjustment mechanism. Tariffs must be adjusted frequently and the process and timing of this adjustment process should be specified.

Appeals and Complaint Procedures

This section must specify the appeals and complaints procedures on the part of providers as well as the insured. They might include:

- going to the court
- use of special appeals committees
- a combination of the two

International Affairs

In the future it may become necessary to include some provisions for dealing with overseas health insurance agencies for entitlement to services provided overseas.

Administrative Organization of the Health Insurance System

In this chapter rules can be laid down about:

- the organizational structure of the health insurance agency;
- the prerogatives of the MOH in appointing the board or the director of the agency;
- the obligation to produce a period (year or quarterly) general and financial account of the activities, revenues and expenditures of the health insurance fund;
- the way health insurance system should execute its mandated authority; and

- the reporting requirements to the MOH and specification of decisions requiring approval from the MOH and others that can be delegated to management.

Implementation

This section should describe the timing and process of implementing the various chapters and articles of the regulation. The implementation schedule could be tied to the execution or completion of other conditions, for example:

- financial development (availability of funds for health insurance, or establishment of health insurance as an independent agency)
- the restructuring of the service delivery system
- the passage of other laws that have an impact on the health insurance fund, e.g., human resource planning and regulation; the planning and licensing of facilities; the quality-assurance issues, etc.

PREREQUISITES TO THE IMPLEMENTATION OF THE LEGISLATIVE SYSTEM FOR HEALTH INSURANCE

Before implementing a new regulation on health insurance, the PA and the MOH should pay particular attention to the following:

- improving the performance of the present providers
- strengthening the information systems, inside the institutions, between the providers and between the MOH (health insurance agency) and providers
- improving the contribution collection mechanism
- strengthening efforts to prevent fraud (unauthorized use of the provisions without payment of contributions or copayment)
- enhancing the capacities of the MOH to formulate policies and evaluate their impact
- strengthening the capabilities of the MOH in reviewing and evaluating the quality and efficiency of the providers, including private providers
- evaluating and revising the copayment system. One of the short-term options is to introduce copayments for emergency care and hospitalizations to promote greater use of the primary health care services. Subsequently, copayments per bed-day could be considered.

PRIVATE HEALTH INSURANCE

The opportunities for private insurers to offer private health insurance and the need for the population to use it will be influenced by the extension of the coverage: if everybody has to be in compulsory insurance for a well-defined package of a reasonable quality, then there will be no incentive to buy a private insurance policy for the same package. In such a situation there will be only a need for supplementary insurance (covering services not enlisted in the public health insurance system or the more luxury variant of the health insurance service as for example a one bed room in an hospital) Such a supplementary private insurance can not be avoided, not even by prohibiting it in the territories: one simply can buy it abroad. However in order to prevent any problems (financial loss) at the side of the insurers as well as the insured the PA must be clear in stating its long-term objectives towards private health insurance and universal coverage.

In the short run it seems even more important to regulate the private providers to avoid a two tier system: a luxury one for the well to do and an old fashioned, less equipped and less friendly system for the average Palestinian. A proper licensing system towards the private providers must be developed and maintained. In this licensing mechanism can be specified the kind of services to be offered and requirements for the facilities (buildings and equipment) in stating minimum and maximum levels. The present way of subcontracting the a limited number of private providers can be extended to the other private and NGO providers insofar as they are required to meet the service needs of the health insurance beneficiaries.

Appendix 14: UPDATED SELECTED POPULATION AND FINANCIAL INFORMATION

Table A 14.1: Selected Figures from Last Population Census

	Total
Total Population (GWB)	3,100,000
Total Population abroad	320,000
Holding ID abroad	
West Bank	248,000
Gaza	76,000
Jerusalem (inside boarders)	210,000
Jerusalem (out side boarders)	113,000
No. of Families GWB	406,896
No of Families in West Bank	262,373
No of Families in Gaza	144,523
Average family size	6.4
West Bank	6.1
Gaza	6.9

Health Insurance

Table A 14.2: No of Insured Families during 1997

Item	No of Insured Families	Total No of Families	Coverage %
Gaza	89,200	144,523	62%
West Bank	108,517	262,373	41%
Police Families	30,000		
Total GWB	227,819		48%

Table A 14.3: Total Revenues from Health Insurance

Type	Revenues (US$ million)
Health insurance revenue	31
Social welfare revenue	5
Police families revenue	3.5
Other revenues	10.5
Grand Total	**50**

Table A 14.4: Detailed Financial Statement of NGO and Private Hospitals & Medical Centers within the PA territories paid by the PA during 1997

No	Hospitals & Medical Centers	Amount
1	Arab Care	183,228
2	Khalid Abu Hospital	103,546
3	Son John Hospital	273,411
4	El-Awda Hospital	23,885
5	Khalil Abu Raia Hospital	166,564
6	Mar Yousif Hospital	38,899
7	Augesta Vectoria Hospital	45,614
8	Gaza Diagnostic Center	206,602
9	El-Wafa Rehabilitation Center	243,550
10	Nablus-Patient Friendship Association	2,980
11	Women's Union Hospital	6,249
12	Prince Basma Association	22,637
13	Islamic Solidarity Center	11,445
14	Artificial Limb Center	66,323
15	Mute Children Society	90,951
16	Medical Technology Company	576
17	Med.-Lab Center	54,568
18	Physical Handicapped Society	5387
19	Beit Lahem Society	67,746
20	El-Bait El-Samed Society	3,356
21	Cerebral Pulsy Center	26,970
22	El-Engely Hospital	2,086
23	Mohamed Ali El-Mohtaseb Hospital	114,306
24	El-Amal Center	896
25	El-Naser Optics	3,101
26	Handicapped Care Society - Gaza	11,335
27	Ahli Arab Hospital - Center	442
28	Al-Qudes Medical Center	37,469
29	Al-Catholic Center - WB	764
30	Makased Benevolent Society	282,121
31	Gaza - Patient friendship Association	33,126
Grand Total		**2,166,133**

Table A 14.5: Hospital Data in Governmental Hospitals in Palestine, 1996

Hospital	No of Bed	Discharge	Deaths	Operations Minor	Major	Births	Days of care	Bed Occupancy (%)	Average length of stay (days)	Out patient Clinic visits
West Bank										
Jenin	55	12,435	180	1,575	1,082	4,583	23,667	117.6	1.9	44,763
Tulkarm	64	8,418	159	928	408	1,929	18,800	80.3	2.2	45,866
Nablus	86	7,340	361	*	*	*	21,867	69.5	3.0	47,191
Rafidiha	138	16,573	138	2,855	1,276	7,863	41,678	82.5	2.5	78,352
Ramallah	142	11,501	304	4,562	1,649	2,581	43,301	83.3	3.8	103,465
Beit Jala	70	6,390	115	1,029	811	1,830	21,085	82.3	3.3	66,745
Jericho	50	3,133	25	499	381	557	9,001	49.2	2.9	33,114
Hebron	103	16,804	182	2,236	2,170	5,435	38,401	101.9	2.3	111,907
Kamal Psychiatric Hosp.	320	571	4	*	*	*	127,823	109.1	223.9	3,366
Gaza Strip										
Shifa	402	36,743	848	3,907	7,744	9,811	121,591	82.9	3.3	148,368
Khan-younis	213	24,182	336	6,931	2,989	6,073	65,200	83.7	2.7	49,100
Pediatric	105	10.39	307	*	*	*	31,926	93.3	3.1	8,219
Opthamalic	31	1,751	0	10,301	1,091	*	6,990	61.8	4.0	67.667
Psychiatric	34	602	0	*	*	*	10,140	81.7	16.8	24.922

Table A 14.6: MOH Revenues ($000)

	H. Insurance	Other Revenues	Total Revenues	MOH Expenses	Coverage %
1996					
Palestine	22,008	9,120	31,128	89,545	34.8
West Bank	12,563	5,824	18,387		
Gaza	9,445	3,296	12,741		
1997					
Palestine	31,014	10,041	41,055	89,448	45.0
West Bank	18,469	6,097	24,566		
Gaza	12,545	3,944	16,489		

Social Welfare Insurance: $5,000
Police Families Medical Services $3,500

Total MOH Revenues in 1997 $49,555 million   55%

Table A 14.7: Households Contribution (1995-1997)

Year	voluntary	Compulsory	Workers	Contract	Soc. Welf	Total
1995						
Palestine	24813	31815	20713	19157	27190	123688
West Bank	9275	19331	8122	9931	12181	58840
Gaza	15538	12484	12591	9226	15009	64848
1996						
Palestine	33136	37975	23559	33927	32315	160912
West Bank	14976	23589	8918	19750	16573	83806
Gaza	18160	14386	14641	14177	15742	77106
1997						
Palestine	36023	45542	28878	47975	39391	197809
West Bank	16919	28571	11992	30151	20884	108517
Gaza	19104	16971	16886	17824	18507	89292

1997

Area	Population	Households	Ins. Household	Coverage %
Palestine	2.89	406896	197809	48
West Bank	1.79	262373	108517	41
Gaza	1.1	144523	89292	62

Distributors of World Bank Publications

Prices and credit terms vary from country to country. Consult your local distributor before placing an order.

ARGENTINA
Oficina del Libro Internacional
Av. Cordoba 1877
1120 Buenos Aires
Tel: (54 1) 815-8354

AUSTRALIA, FIJI, PAPUA NEW GUINEA, SOLOMON ISLANDS, VANUATU, AND SAMOA
D.A. Information Services
648 Whitehorse Road
Mitcham 3132
Victoria
Tel: (61) 3 9210 7777

AUSTRIA
Gerold and Co.
Weihburggasse 26
A-1011 Wien
Tel: (43 1) 512-47-31-0

BANGLADESH
Micro Industries Development
Assistance Society (MIDAS)
House 5, Road 16
Dhanmondi R/Area
Dhaka 1209
Tel: (880 2) 326427

BELGIUM
Jean De Lannoy
Av. du Roi 202
1060 Brussels
Tel: (32 2) 538-5169

BRAZIL
Publicações Técnicas Internacionais Ltda.
Rua Peixoto Gomide, 209
01409 Sao Paulo, SP.
Tel: (55 11) 259-6644

CANADA
Renouf Publishing Co. Ltd.
5369 Canotek Road
Ottawa, Ontario K1J 9J3
Tel: (613) 745-2665

CHINA
China Financial & Economic
Publishing House
8, Da Fo Si Dong Jie
Beijing
Tel: (86 10) 6333-8257

China Book Import Centre
P.O. Box 2825
Beijing

COLOMBIA
Infoenlace Ltda.
Carrera 6 No. 51-21
Apartado Aereo 34270
Santafé de Bogotá, D.C.
Tel: (571) 285-2798

COTE D'IVOIRE
Center d'Edition et de Diffusion
Africaines (CEDA)
04 B.P. 541
Abidjan 04
Tel: (225) 24 6510;24 6511

CYPRUS
Center for Applied Research
Cyprus College
6, Diogenes Street, Engomi
P.O. Box 2006
Nicosia
Tel: (357 2) 44-1730

CZECH REPUBLIC
USIS, NIS Prodejna
Havelkova 22
130 00 Prague 3
Tel: (420 2) 2423 1486

DENMARK
SamfundsLitteratur
Rosenoerns Allé 11
DK-1970 Frederiksberg C
Tel: (45 31) 351942

ECUADOR
Libri Mundi
Libreria Internacional
P.O. Box 17-01-3029
Juan Leon Mera 851
Quito
Tel: (593 2) 521-606; (593 2) 544-185

CODEU
Ruiz de Castilla 763, Edif. Expocolor
Primer piso, Of. #2
Quito
Tel/Fax: (593 2) 507-383; 253-091

EGYPT, ARAB REPUBLIC OF
Al Ahram Distribution Agency
Al Galaa Street
Cairo
Tel: (20 2) 578-6083

The Middle East Observer
41, Sherif Street
Cairo
Tel: (20 2) 393-9732
Fax: (20 2) 393-9732

FINLAND
Akateeminen Kirjakauppa
P.O. Box 128
FIN-00101 Helsinki
Tel: (358 0) 121 4418

FRANCE
World Bank Publications
66, avenue d'Iéna
75116 Paris
Tel: (33 1) 40-69-30-56/57

GERMANY
UNO-Verlag
Poppelsdorfer Allee 55
53115 Bonn
Tel: (49 228) 949020

GHANA
Epp Books Services
P.O. Box 44
TUC
Accra

GREECE
Papasotiriou S.A.
35, Stournara Str.
106 82 Athens
Tel: (30 1) 364-1826

HAITI
Culture Diffusion
5, Rue Capois
C.P. 257
Port-au-Prince
Tel: (509) 23 9260

HONG KONG, MACAO
Asia 2000 Ltd.
Sales & Circulation Department
302 Seabird House
22-28 Wyndham Street, Central
Hong Kong
Tel: (852) 2530-1409

HUNGARY
Euro Info Service
Margitszgeti Europa Haz
H-1138 Budapest
Tel: (36 1) 350 80 24, 350 80 25

INDIA
Allied Publishers Ltd.
751 Mount Road
Madras - 600 002
Tel: (91 44) 852-3938

INDONESIA
Pt. Indira Limited
Jalan Borobudur 20
P.O. Box 181
Jakarta 10320
Tel: (62 21) 390-4290

IRAN
Ketab Sara Co. Publishers
Khaled Eslamboli Ave., 6th Street
Delafrooz Alley No. 8
P.O. Box 15745-733
Tehran 15117
Tel: (98 21) 8717819; 8716104

Kowkab Publishers
P.O. Box 19575-511
Tehran
Tel: (98 21) 258-3723

IRELAND
Government Supplies Agency
Oifig an tSolathair
4-5 Harcourt Road
Dublin 2
Tel: (353 1) 661-3111

ISRAEL
Yozmot Literature Ltd.
P.O. Box 56055
3 Yohanan Hasandlar Street
Tel Aviv 61560
Tel: (972 3) 5285-397

R.O.Y. International
PO Box 13056
Tel Aviv 61130
Tel: (972 3) 5461423

Palestinian Authority/Middle East
Index Information Services
P.O.B. 19502 Jerusalem
Tel: (972 2) 6271219

ITALY
Licosa Commissionaria Sansoni SPA
Via Duca Di Calabria, 1/1
Casella Postale 552
50125 Firenze
Tel: (55) 645-415

JAMAICA
Ian Randle Publishers Ltd.
206 Old Hope Road, Kingston 6
Tel: 876-927-2085

JAPAN
Eastern Book Service
3-13 Hongo 3-chome, Bunkyo-ku
Tokyo 113
Tel: (81 3) 3818-0861

KENYA
Africa Book Service (E.A.) Ltd.
Quaran House, Mfangano Street
P.O. Box 45245
Nairobi
Tel: (254 2) 223 641

KOREA, REPUBLIC OF
Daejon Trading Co. Ltd.
P.O. Box 34, Youida, 706 Seoun Bldg
44-6 Youido-Dong, Yeongchengo-Ku
Seoul
Tel: (82 2) 785-1631/4

LEBANON
Librairie du Liban
P.O. Box 11-9232
Beirut
Tel: (961 9) 217 944

MALAYSIA
University of Malaya Cooperative
Bookshop, Limited
P.O. Box 1127
Jalan Pantai Baru
59700 Kuala Lumpur
Tel: (60 3) 756-5000

MEXICO
INFOTEC
Av. San Fernando No. 37
Col. Toriello Guerra
14050 Mexico, D.F.
Tel: (52 5) 624-2800

Mundi-Prensa Mexico S.A. de C.V.
c/Rio Panuco, 141-Colonia Cuauhtemoc
06500 Mexico, D.F.
Tel: (52 5) 533-5658

NEPAL
Everest Media International Services
(P) Ltd.
GPO Box 5443
Kathmandu
Tel: (977 1) 472 152

NETHERLANDS
De Lindeboom/InOr-Publikaties
P.O. Box 202, 7480 AE Haaksbergen
Tel: (31 53) 574-0004

NEW ZEALAND
EBSCO NZ Ltd.
Private Mail Bag 99914
New Market
Auckland
Tel: (64 9) 524-8119

NIGERIA
University Press Limited
Three Crowns Building Jericho
Private Mail Bag 5095
Ibadan
Tel: (234 22) 41-1356

NORWAY
NIC Info A/S
Book Department, Postboks 6512
Etterstad
N-0606 Oslo
Tel: (47 22) 97-4500

PAKISTAN
Mirza Book Agency
65, Shahrah-e-Quaid-e-Azam
Lahore 54000
Tel: (92 42) 735 3601

Oxford University Press
5 Bangalore Town
Sharae Faisal
PO Box 13033
Karachi-75350
Tel: (92 21) 446307

Pak Book Corporation
Aziz Chambers 21, Queen's Road
Lahore
Tel: (92 42) 636 3222; 636 0885

PERU
Editorial Desarrollo SA
Apartado 3824, Lima 1
Tel: (51 14) 285380

PHILIPPINES
International Booksource Center Inc.
1127-A Antipolo St, Barangay,
Venezuela
Makati City
Tel: (63 2) 896 6501; 6505; 6507

POLAND
International Publishing Service
Ul. Piekna 31/37
00-677 Warzawa
Tel: (48 2) 628-6089

PORTUGAL
Livraria Portugal
Apartado 2681, Rua Do Carmo 70-74
1200 Lisbon
Tel: (1) 347-4982

ROMANIA
Compani De Librarii Bucuresti S.A.
Str. Lipscani no. 26, sector 3
Bucharest
Tel: (40 1) 613 9645

RUSSIAN FEDERATION
Isdatelstvo <Ves Mir>
9a, Kolpachniy Pereulok
Moscow 101831
Tel: (7 095) 917 87 49

SINGAPORE; TAIWAN, CHINA MYANMAR; BRUNEI
Hemisphere Publication Services
41 Kallang Pudding Road #04-03
Golden Wheel Building
Singapore 349316
Tel: (65) 741-5166

SLOVENIA
Gospodarski Vestnik Publishing Group
Dunajska cesta 5
1000 Ljubljana
Tel: (386 61) 133 83 47; 132 12 30

SOUTH AFRICA, BOTSWANA
For single titles:
Oxford University Press Southern Africa
Vasco Boulevard, Goodwood
P.O. Box 12119, N1 City 7463
Cape Town
Tel: (27 21) 595 4400

For subscription orders:
International Subscription Service
P.O. Box 41095
Craighall
Johannesburg 2024
Tel: (27 11) 880-1448

SPAIN
Mundi-Prensa Libros, S.A.
Castello 37
28001 Madrid
Tel: (34 1) 431-3399

Mundi-Prensa Barcelona
Consell de Cent, 391
08009 Barcelona
Tel: (34 3) 488-3492

SRI LANKA, THE MALDIVES
Lake House Bookshop
100, Sir Chittampalam Gardiner
Mawatha
Colombo 2
Tel: (94 1) 32105

SWEDEN
Wennergren-Williams AB
P.O. Box 1305
S-171 25 Solna
Tel: (46 8) 705-97-50

SWITZERLAND
Librairie Payot Service Institutionnel
Côtes-de-Montbenon 30
1002 Lausanne
Tel: (1 21) 341-3229

ADECO Van Diemen
Editions Techniques
Ch. de Lacuez 41
CH1807 Blonay
Tel: (1 21) 943 2673

THAILAND
Central Books Distribution
306 Silom Road
Bangkok 10500
Tel: (66 2) 235-5400

TRINIDAD & TOBAGO AND THE CARRIBBEAN
Systematics Studies Ltd.
St. Augustine Shopping Center
Eastern Main Road, St. Augustine
Trinidad & Tobago, West Indies
Tel: (868) 645-8466

UGANDA
Gustro Ltd.
PO Box 9997, Madhvani Building
Plot 16/4 Jinja Rd.
Kampala
Tel: (256 41) 251 467

UNITED KINGDOM
Microinfo Ltd.
P.O. Box 3, Alton, Hampshire GU34 2PG
England
Tel: (44 1420) 86848

The Stationery Office
51 Nine Elms Lane
London SW8 5DR
Tel: (44 171) 873-8400

VENEZUELA
Tecni-Ciencia Libros, S.A.
Centro Cuidad Comercial Tamanco
Nivel C2, Caracas
Tel: (58 2) 959 5547; 5035; 0016

ZAMBIA
University Bookshop, University of
Zambia
Great East Road Campus
P.O. Box 32379
Lusaka
Tel: (260 1) 252 576

ZIMBABWE
Academic and Baobab Books (Pvt.) Ltd.
4 Conald Road, Graniteside
P.O. Box 567
Harare
Tel: 263 4 755035

5/29/98